The Yoga Sutras of Patanjali

RANJIT CHAUDHRI

FiNGERPRINT!

Published by
FINGERPRINT!
An imprint of Prakash Books India Pvt. Ltd

113/A, Darya Ganj,
New Delhi-110 002
Email: info@prakashbooks.com/sales@prakashbooks.com

Fingerprint Publishing
@FingerprintP
@fingerprintpublishingbooks
www.fingerprintpublishing.com

ISBN: 978 93 6214 275 7

DEDICATION

To Maharishi Patanjali, with gratitude,
for showing us the way.

CONTENTS

INTRODUCTION

We spend most of our time trying to increase our wealth and improve our standard of living. Greater wealth certainly makes our lives more comfortable and gives us the freedom to do more things, but it does not remove our suffering or bring about fulfillment. That can only come about through a higher level of consciousness. For this reason, Patanjali's *Yoga Sutras* is one of the preeminent spiritual texts of the world. It was written mainly to show us how to raise our consciousness and be liberated. It also answers some of life's fundamental questions—Why are we here? What is the purpose of this world? What causes our suffering? How does life work? Patanjali lists the five afflictions that cause suffering and explains how to remove them. He displays a very deep understanding of how life works. He explains the karmic process that governs our life and how we can set it aside. There is profound wisdom and also practical wisdom that we can apply in our lives. Patanjali groups all the people we may meet into four categories and shows us how to interact with each type of person.

Maharishi Patanjali is considered the father of yoga. He was not the founder of yoga. The founder of yoga is Lord Shiva, who first taught yoga to the seven sages (the *Saptarishis*) on the south face of Mount Kailash (in present-day Tibet) over 10,000 years ago. Patanjali organized yoga and made it more systematic. He grouped some of the important practices of yoga into eight limbs. He explained the importance of each of the eight limbs and how they bring about our liberation.

The word *Yoga* means union. It also means to join or to yoke. Yoga is about the union of the individual with the Divine. The word *Sutra* literally means thread. It is meant to contain the essence of something. From a thread, you can stitch many types of cloth. Similarly, from a Sutra, you can add and explain the truth or message it is conveying. A master was supposed to explain each Sutra in greater detail to his disciples. It is something like an equation or formula, which you expand upon. There is a significant amount of theory behind an equation. An equation is a concise essence of something. A sutra is just like that. The message it contains needs to be expanded and explained. The reason some ancient texts were written in sutras was for practical purposes. There was no method of writing and recording texts in those days. Texts were memorized and passed down orally from generation to generation. The only way a text could be memorized accurately was if it was brief. Hence, the necessity of conveying knowledge through sutras. A sutra is usually not even a complete sentence. Sometimes, it may just be three words. Occasionally, this creates problems while translating, as a few different options may be possible.

The *Yoga Sutras* consists of 196 sutras, divided into four chapters. Each chapter has the word *Pāda* in its title. *Pāda* means chapter or quarter. For example, the first chapter is titled *Samādhi Pāda.* This means "Chapter on Samadhi" or "Quarter on Samadhi".

The first chapter is on the state of *Samadhi,* which is a state very close to liberation. Patanjali explains some ways of reaching this state. He also defines yoga and liberation. He examines in some detail the activities of the mind and how we can still it. His understanding of how the mind works is brilliant. It is far deeper than modern-day psychology. He exhibits a comprehensive understanding of the way the mind functions and the means to control it.

The second chapter is titled *Spiritual Practice.* It can be divided into two equal parts. In the first part, Patanjali discusses Kriya yoga, the afflictions that cause suffering and the means to remove them, and the Law of Karma. He also explains the purpose of the physical world and how it progressively comes into being. This part of the chapter discusses some of the philosophy behind yoga and the process of liberation.

In the second part of the chapter, Patanjali explains the eight limbs of yoga and the benefits of practicing each limb. This is the part that Patanjali has been known for—for organizing yoga into eight limbs.

The third chapter is titled *Spiritual Powers.* It explains the last three limbs of yoga and the spiritual powers that may arise when they are practiced together. Patanjali explains the whole gamut of powers that one may acquire and how they can hinder one's liberation. Finally, at the end of the chapter, he explains what is required for our enlightenment.

The fourth chapter is titled *Liberation.* It discusses the law of Karma and the philosophy behind yoga. Finally, the chapter discusses our Liberation and the way to get there.

The chapter titles are a broad guideline to the content of the chapter. The chapters contain information on a lot more subjects than what their titles suggest. There is also an overlap in the topics covered in the chapters. For example, spiritual practice is discussed in all four chapters, not just in the second chapter that has it as its title. Similarly, Samadhi and liberation are also discussed in all four chapters.

There is an interesting legend about Patanjali's birth. *Adi Shesha,* the king of the serpents, was blessed by Lord Shiva and informed by him that he would take birth as a human. At the time, there was a pious lady called *Gonika,* who was praying fervently to Lord Shiva for a son, with her palms open. Adi Shesha fell into her palms and took the form of a human. This is why he was given the name Patanjali. Patanjali is made up of two words, *Pat* which means to descend or to fall, and *anjali* which means to have your hands open, placed side by side. Adi Shesha literally fell into the palms of Gonika. Patanjali is also called *Gonikaputra,* which means, "son of Gonika".

In addition to the *Yoga Sutras* Patanjali wrote a book on grammar (*Mahabhashya*) and medicine (*Charakapratisanskrita*). In his book on grammar, he states that he resided in Kashmir for a few years. Patanjali is believed to have consecrated the *linga* at the Chidambaram temple in Tamil Nadu. Some Western scholars believe that there are three different Patanjalis who authored these three texts. The Indian tradition maintains that it is the same Patanjali, who authored all three books. Patanjali had an excellent command of the Sanskrit language. He is very economical with his words. Not a single word is wasted. In the 196 sutras, he uses a verb only on three or four occasions and still conveys his message clearly. His style of instruction is straight to the point, matter of fact, and concise. He uses words that precisely describe the subject.

Patanjali is sometimes depicted as half-man, half-snake. The top of his body is human, and the base of his body is shown as a snake. Part of the reason for this depiction is the legend about his birth but there is also a deeper meaning to this. The snake has special significance in yoga. It is used to depict the dormant energy within us, called *Kundalini*. A snake is very still. We only notice it when it starts moving. Similarly, *Kundalini,* our dormant energy, remains unnoticed by most people as it has not been awakened. It is only noticed when it is activated and starts rising. When *Kundalini* reaches the top of our heads, we are liberated. Patanjali's depiction as half-man, half-snake is to show that he is fully liberated. His *Kundalini* has risen, and he is one with God.

When were the *Yoga Sutras* written? There are two broad dates given by the scholars: 9th–10th century BC or 2nd–5th century BC. The style of writing is ancient. The meaning of some of the words used in the *Yoga Sutras* seem to have changed later, which is why a few of the sutras are difficult to translate. The meanings of some words get altered over time and the dictionary usually emphasizes their latter date meaning. The *Yoga Sutras* may very well belong to the earlier 9–10th century BC period.

At one time, the *Yoga Sutras* were very popular in India. Their popularity peaked between the 7th and 12th centuries and they were translated into 40 Indian regional languages. Then, from the 12th century, after the Islamic invasions of India, the text disappeared for a few centuries until it was revived by Swami Vivekananda in the late 19th century.

What is the philosophy behind the *Yoga Sutras?* What school of thought does it belong to? Some commentators believe that the *Yoga Sutras* are similar to the *Samkhya* philosophy. There are some similarities with *Samkhya,* especially with a few of the terms used. However, there are some significant differences too. *Samkhya* is an atheistic philosophy and has no God. In the *Yoga Sutras,* God is prominently mentioned in a few of the sutras. *Samkhya* is also a dualistic philosophy. The *Yoga Sutras* as explained below, is non-dualistic. *Samkhya* does not contain any reference to the eight-limbed practice of yoga, given in the *Yoga Sutras.* The *Yoga Sutras* has a lot in common with the *Bhagavad Gita* (especially Chapters Two and Six) and with parts of Buddhism. Sutra 15 of the second chapter is very similar to the first of the four Noble Truths in Buddhism; about the suffering we experience in life. Patanjali, himself, does not mention any other text or philosophy in the *Yoga Sutras.* Instead, he gives the philosophy behind yoga in Chapters Two and Four.

More importantly, does the text belong to the philosophy of non-dualism or dualism? There are two great philosophical, spiritual traditions in India: non-dualism and dualism. The dualistic tradition maintains that the physical world, called Nature, is a separate entity from individual souls. There are multiple individual souls which are bound in Nature. Freeing the individual soul from Nature is liberation. Non-dualism states that only God exists. Everything and everyone are part of God. God is consciousness, and the physical world is created by the energy of consciousness. The fact that we appear separate from each other is an illusion. Individual souls are always part of the Universal Soul (God). Experiencing or realizing our oneness with God is called self-realization, or liberation.

Patanjali starts by being dualistic. He mentions in Chapter One that God is a special soul not bound by the karmic process. He seems to imply that God is separate from the individual souls following the karmic process. However, in Chapter Two, Patanjali suddenly shifts to non-dualism. His description of ignorance and liberation is completely non-dualistic. In Chapter Four, he delves further into non-dualism. The last sutra of Chapter Four describes the state of liberation. The description is completely non-dualistic. Patanjali is very clever with his usage of words. As mentioned earlier, his words aptly describe the subject it is used for. For example, *asmitā* which means "I-ness', is used for the ego. He also uses the word *Seer* for the soul. Seer is a great way to describe the soul. Our soul is consciousness; it is awareness, or the witness within us, and has far greater perception than our mind. Seer is a perfect way to describe the soul. Patanjali uses the word *Kaivalya* for liberation. *Kaivalya* means absolute unity, or absolute oneness. It is derived from the word *Kevala*, which means one, sole, alone, only. It is a very non-dualistic word for liberation. Patanjali could have used other words for liberation but chooses one that aptly describes liberation in a non-dualistic way. In fact, he names the fourth chapter, *Kaivalya Pāda*—Chapter on Liberation. He not only discusses liberation but also the philosophy of non-dualism in this chapter.

Most Sanskrit words have more than one possible meaning in English. In some cases, Patanjali is using more than one meaning for a word. In these instances, both meanings are given so that the reader can understand precisely what Patanjali is trying to convey.

The four chapters have been translated with commentary. At the end of the book, the sutras have been repeated without commentary, so you may read it and draw your wisdom from it.

Some of the wisdom contained in this text will jolt you. It will make you look at life in a completely different way. It may even turn your world upside down. Part of the message given here; you may have heard earlier. This is because this is a text that has influenced and shaped the culture of India for centuries. In any event, this is a text that may impact you deeply. It has the potential to open your life to a completely new dimension—a dimension beyond the physical world of our sense organs.

CHAPTER ONE

SAMĀDHI PĀDA

SAMADHI

1

Atha yogānuśāsanam

Now, instructions on yoga.

If you are satisfied and happy with your life, you really do not need to read any further. This is a book for those longing for more—more peace, more joy, more clarity in life, and more enlightenment. You may be tired of the suffering you are experiencing and are looking for a way out. You may be fed up with your life situation and may want answers on how life works. Or, you may have practiced some yoga and may want to know more about what yoga has to offer. Or, you may simply have a desire to be enlightened. You have seen all the material world has to offer and have decided that this does not satisfy you. Becoming enlightened becomes your overwhelming desire and the focus of your life. If you fit into any of these categories, then you have come to the right place.

2

Yogaś citta-vṛtti-nirodhaḥ

Stilling the activities of the mind is yoga.

Patanjali wastes no time and gets straight to the point. This sutra and the next are amongst the most important sutras in the text. The rest of the text is set up to explain these two sutras.

Yoga literally means "union". It is the union of the individual with the Divine or of the human being with God. How does one achieve this union? By stilling the activities of the mind. Patanjali explains in great detail later in the text how this is to be achieved.

Our educational system teaches us about the physical sciences and the social sciences. Physical sciences such as Physics, Chemistry and Biology explain the physical, chemical, and biological properties of objects found in the external world. The social sciences, such as economics and political science, teach us about the marketplace, our political systems, and our interactions with each other. However, there is very little taught to us about our mind, our body, and our life energies. The human body and mind are the most complex living organism in the planet. And we are taught very little about how to use them.

Yoga, on the other hand, can be called an inner science. It is the science for our liberation. It explains to us in great detail how we can use our mind, body and life energies to transcend our mundane existence and achieve liberation.

To achieve liberation, we need to still the activities of the mind. The word *nirodha* has been used here. *Nirodha* literally means to control, check, restrain, or destroy. Normally, our mind is uncontrolled. We are continuously thinking, and we have very little control over this endless stream of thoughts. Yoga is the science of stilling the activities of the mind.

3

Tadā draṣṭuḥ svarūpe 'vasthānam

Then, the Seer abides in its own nature.

Patanjali uses an interesting word for the soul. He calls it the "Seer". It is a very accurate description of the soul. Our soul is pure consciousness, or awareness. It is the witness within us that is aware of all our activities. In yoga, we usually refer to the soul as the Self, or the Seer.

When the mind is stilled, the Seer abides by its own nature. The mind is like a layer of dirt over a mirror. When there is dirt on a mirror, you cannot see yourself clearly. When the dirt is removed, one can see one's Self clearly. The Seer's nature is awareness and bliss. When the mind is active, there is no awareness or joy. Most of us live mundane lives. We do not experience the joy of the Self because our mind is uncontrolled. When we start stilling the mind, we experience more peace, more awareness, and more joy. When the mind is completely still, we experience the bliss of our true nature—*the Seer abides in its own nature.*

We sometimes use the phrase, "peace of mind". Peace is actually from the mind, not of the mind. We can be truly peaceful only when we are free of the mind, or in a state without the active mind. Ramana Maharshi used to say that happiness is born of peace. Peace arises only when there is no disturbance of thoughts in the mind. He said unless we annihilate the mind, we cannot gain peace or happiness.

4

Vṛtti-sārūpyam itaratra

Otherwise, one identifies with the activities of the mind.

Our ego is a constituent of the mind. It is our identification with name and form. It is our sense of separate identity. When the mind is active, we identify with the body and the individual person that we are. We further identify with our race, our gender, our nationality, and our religion. We bond with or feel a sense of closeness with other members or our race, nationality, or religion. It is these limited identities that breed violence and conflict. In ancient India, children were taught to repeat, "*Aham Brahmasmi*", every day. *Aham Brahmasmi* literally means, "I am Brahman (God)", or "I am Divine". This was taught to children to break their limited identifications with their body, race, religion, and nationality, and emphasize their eternal oneness with God.

When we are in a state of awareness, we identify with our Self, or our soul. When the mind is active, we lose our self-awareness and identify with our mind and body, and our individuality.

5

Vṛttayaḥ pañcatayyaḥ kliṣṭākliṣṭāḥ

There are five types of activities of the mind, and these are either painful or pain-free.

Patanjali now proceeds to describe the various activities of the mind. Some of these activities cause pain and some do not.

6

Pramāṇa-viparyaya-vikalpa-nidrā-smṛtayaḥ

They are right beliefs, wrong beliefs, imagination, sleep, and memory.

There are other spiritual texts that also tell us to still the mind in order to experience liberation. However, Patanjali goes into more detail. He divides the activities of the mind into five categories. The mind creates beliefs. These beliefs may be right or wrong. It imagines a variety of things, it sleeps, and it thinks of the past (memory).

7

Pratyakṣānumānāgamāḥ pramāṇāni

The sources of right beliefs are direct experience, inference, and authoritative scriptures.

A belief is our notion or idea about something, or about how things work. There are three ways of arriving at a belief. The first is direct experience. We touch ice and we know it is cold. From our experience we can say that ice is cold. We can also arrive at a belief through inference. We see lightning and we know it is going to rain. This is because lightning is associated with an electric storm. Or, by smelling certain foods, we can infer they may not be fit to consume. Stale food emits a certain smell. Finally, we can arrive at a belief through authoritative scriptures. These are not just any scriptures but scriptures that are reliable and are an authority in their subject. The knowledge found in these texts is the knowledge given by others who have arrived at it through their own work. For example, we learn from books that the earth is round. We may not have experienced this ourselves by traveling to outer space, but from books, we see photographs and scientific reasoning for the earth being round.

8

Viparyayo mithyā-jñānam
atad-rūpa-pratiṣṭham

Wrong beliefs are false knowledge that is not based on the true nature of something.

Sometimes the mind creates beliefs that are incorrect and devoid of reality. A few of these beliefs even create fear in the minds of those holding them. Most people are scared of death. This is usually because of fear of the unknown. Some believe it is the end of them and they will cease to exist. This belief is completely incorrect. We are not the body; we are the soul. It is the soul that breathes life into the body. The body dying is not the end of our existence. Our soul is imperishable and lives forever. As the *Spanda Karikas* (Verses 14–16) explains so eloquently:

Two are found to exist here, called the Creator and the created. Among them, created matter is subject to decay, but the Creator is imperishable.

Looking at created matter dissolving into the Whole, examine carefully what is being destroyed here. At the time of his death, an ignorant man thinks, "I will cease to exist."

But the Being within us, who is the abode of the quality of omniscience, cannot be destroyed. Due to lack of knowledge of his other Self, a man believes, sooner or later, he may cease to exist.

9

Śabda-jñānānupātī vastu-śūnyo vikalpaḥ

Knowledge resulting from words that are devoid of reality is imagination.

Imagination is an activity the mind spends a lot of time on. It is something we are doing constantly. We imagine ourselves talking to certain people or, in certain situations, interacting with other people in a particular way. This happens more frequently when something goes wrong in our life or if someone has disturbed us. Then, the mind keeps thinking of various negative events that could happen in our life as a consequence of whatever has gone wrong. For example, if we lose our job, we start thinking about how we will pay our bills, look after our children, and so on. Sometimes, the mind starts imagining the worst, that we may never get another job again, or we may have to sell our house. Imagination is the activity of the mind that can cause suffering. This is looked at in greater detail later on.

In a crisis, it becomes a challenge to still the mind. But it becomes necessary in those very situations to calm the mind. From a calm mind great ideas flow, ideas that could be the solution to the very problems we are facing. When we still the mind, we are able to access the wisdom of the soul. This wisdom can be accessed only when the mind is still, not when it is agitated.

10

Abhāva-pratyayālambanā vṛttir nidrā

Sleep is the activity, without the intellect as its foundation.

Patanjali is referring to the state of deep sleep, where there are no dreams. In that state, the mind is quiet, and the intellect is absent. The state of deep sleep is close to the state of enlightenment, in that the mind is still. However, there is one crucial difference—in deep sleep, there is no awareness. In a liberated state, the mind is absent but there is also full awareness.

Patanjali calls sleep an activity of the mind, and it is one of the five activities that need to be stopped. So, what is wrong with sleep, and why should we try and stop it? After all, sleep gives us rest and without sleep we would not be able to function in this world. Sleep is an activity without awareness, and we need to bring in awareness while sleeping. This is not something we can practice while we are working on our liberation. However, a liberated person is aware during all the states of mind. Normally there are three states of mind—the state of wakefulness, the state of sleep with dreams, and the state of deep sleep. There is also a fourth state called *Turiya. Turiya* is a state of enlightenment. When we reach this state, we are aware during all the other three states of wakefulness, dream, and deep sleep.

11

Anubhūta-viṣayāsaṁpramoṣaḥ smṛtiḥ

Past experiences remembered, is memory.

Finally, the fifth activity of the mind is memory. Remembering past experiences of our life, is memory. During the wakeful state, the mind spends most of its time between imagination and memory. We are either imagining various things, or we are living in the past. The movement toward liberation is to spend more time in the present. To be aware and live fully in the present moment, and not in the past or in our imagination. This means paying full attention to the present moment and to whatever life brings us. *Attentiveness is the seed,* as the *Shiva Sutras* state (3.15).

12

Abhyāsa-vairāgyābhyāṁ tan-nirodhaḥ

The activities of the mind are stilled by continuous practice and detachment.

Patanjali has described the five activities of the mind, and he now begins to explain how to control or still the mind. He spends a major part of the next chapter explaining this, but now he focuses on the two most important elements of any spiritual practice—continuous practice and detachment.

Lord Krishna gives a similar advice in the *Bhagavad Gita* (6.35): *Undoubtedly, the restless mind is difficult to control, O mighty armed one. But Arjuna, by continuous practice and detachment, the mind is stilled.*

Interestingly, the *Bhagavad Gita* uses the same words as the *Yoga Sutras*—continuous practice (*abhyāsa*) and detachment (*vairāgya*).

13

Tatra sthitau yatno 'bhyāsaḥ

Of the two, perseverance in effort is continuous practice.

Whatever spiritual practice we choose, unless we persevere in it, we have very little chance of success. Continuous practice means to persevere in our efforts.

14

Sa tu dīrgha-kāla-nairantarya-satkārāsevito dṛḍha-bhūmiḥ

And it becomes firmly established, when it is practiced uninterruptedly for a long time, with care and attention.

Our spiritual practice becomes firmly established, when we practice it continuously without interruption, for a long period of time. We also have to practice it with care and attention. It cannot be something we just do routinely, like brushing our teeth. It has to be done with attention, so that we do it properly. Once it is done properly for a period of time, it brings the results we desire.

15

Dṛṣṭānuśravika-viṣaya-vitṛṣṇasya vaśikāra-saṁjñā vairāgyam

Detachment is that mastered state of consciousness, when one is not desirous of sense objects, whether experienced or heard.

Now, Patanjali explains what he means by detachment. Detachment means not desiring sense objects or pleasures of the senses. We may have experienced these sense objects or heard about them from others. Detachment means not craving these sense objects or pleasures. Sensory detachment is the fifth limb of yoga and Patanjali explains it in further detail at the end of the next chapter.

Why is detachment from objects of sense important for stilling the mind? This is because, without detachment, one is always thinking about sensory pleasures. A lustful man thinks about sex. A person who loves food will think mostly about food. Others think about money and the pleasures it can buy. To still the mind one has to transcend the pleasures of the body. We are not the body and when we are able to go beyond the pleasures the body craves, it becomes possible to control the mind. There is a beautiful meditation in the *Vigyan Bhairava Tantra* (Verse 136) that explains how to use detachment to still the mind:

All contact with pleasure, pain, etc., are through the sense organs. Therefore, one should detach oneself from the senses, turn within, and abide in one's own Self.

16

Tat-paraṁ puruṣa-khyāter guṇa-vaitṛṣṇyam

Following that, due to the perception of the soul, there is freedom from desires for the qualities of nature.

When we persevere in our spiritual practice and make progress in detaching from sensory objects, our mind becomes increasingly still. When the mind starts falling silent, we experience the peace and joy of the soul. Once we have tasted the joy of the soul, the pleasures of the external world no longer interest us. The pleasures of the external world, referred to here as the qualities of nature, are essentially pleasures of the body. The pleasures of the soul are far greater than the pleasures of the body. Once they are experienced, one no longer desires the pleasures of the outside world. Our cravings and our addictions, just fall away.

Sri Ramana Maharshi gave a beautiful example to explain this. He said if a cow continuously strays outside her stall, her owner tempts her to stay inside with fine grass and fodder. At first, she may refuse, but gradually she enjoys being in the stall. After a while, even if she is let loose, she will not stray out of her stall. Similarly, with the mind. Once it finds inner happiness, it will no longer wander outwards, seeking sensory pleasures.

17

Vitarka-vicārānandāsmitānugamāt samprajñātaḥ

By extinguishing thinking, reflection, sensual enjoyment, and egoism, one attains Samprajnata (Samadhi).

The word *Samprajnata* means distinguished, discerned, or to know accurately. Patanjali explains the state of Samadhi later in this chapter. It is a state where the mind is very still, and one is close to liberation. It is a very high level of consciousness. *Samprajnata Samadhi* means we are in a state where we are able to discern or know things accurately. We can make out what is real and what is unreal. We can see past the illusion and experience true reality.

We reach this state by extinguishing thinking, reflection, sensual enjoyment, and egoism. Thinking and reflection are activities of the mind, which need to be stopped. Extinguishing sensual enjoyment doesn't mean we don't enjoy things of the world. It means that there is no addiction or attachment to sensual pleasures. As sutras 12 and 15 explained, detachment from sense objects is necessary for stilling the mind.

Finally, egoism also needs to be extinguished. Patanjali uses a word here, *asmitā,* which has been translated as egoism. *Asmitā* is made up of two words, *asmi* and *tā*. *Asmi* is the first person singular of the verb *as* and means 'I'. *Tā* is a suffix that denotes 'ness'. Therefore, *asmitā* literally means 'I-ness'. The dictionary translates *asmitā* as egoism, which is the meaning that has been used in this translation but the literal meaning 'I-ness', gives you a better description of the ego. The ego is this feeling of individuality (I-ness), where we identify with our body and mind and the individual person that we are. Patanjali asks us to give up the identification with the body. When we are able to do this, we attain *Samprajnata Samadhi.*

18

Virāma-pratyayābhyāsa-pūrvaḥ
saṁskāra-śeṣo 'nyaḥ

Through the continuous practice mentioned earlier, the intellect ceases and only the impressions remain. This is another way.

The continuous practice mentioned earlier was in Sutra 12. Through continuous practice and detachment, the mind is stilled, and one attains Samadhi.

In some of the next few sutras, Patanjali gives us different ways to attain Samadhi. He first gives different methods for attaining Samadhi before he fully explains what Samadhi is.

The impressions are our stock of karma. This is explained in greater detail, later in this chapter.

19

Bhava-pratyayo videha-prakṛti-layānām

Yogis not identified with their bodies, attain this stilled state of being.

Identifying with our body is the cause of our bondage. Nisargadatta Maharaj used to say that liberation is never of the person, it is from the person. One of the most profound spiritual texts to come out of India is the *Ashtavakra Gita*. In its first few verses it makes the remarkable statement that if we set the body aside (stop identifying with the body), and rest in awareness, we will be liberated at once. When we no longer identify with our body, we identify with our Self, which is pure awareness. When we are aware, the mind is automatically still.

Yogis used to practice various meditations to break their identification with the body. The *Vigyan Bhairava Tantra* has a number of them. Verse 48 of that text states:

Consider the skin to be the wall of an empty body with nothing inside. By meditating like this, one reaches a place beyond meditation.

20

Śraddhā-vīrya-smṛti-samādhi-prajñā-pūrvaka itareṣām

For others, Samprajnata Samadhi is preceded by faith, vigour, and remembrance.

To achieve our goal, there has to be an effort from our side. God is there to help us on the way but there is no such thing as a free pass in life. We cannot expect that we will do nothing and God's grace will descend on and liberate us. No, there has to be vigorous and continuous effort from our side. The *Shiva Sutras* state: *vigorous and continuous effort leads to God* (1.5).

Faith is an important component in any spiritual journey. We need to have faith that our spiritual practice will bring results, even though those results may not be immediately evident. Our spiritual practice brings about change within us. Sometimes it may appear that the progress is slow but then suddenly, one day we may awaken to another dimension of existence. Ramana Maharshi explained to his disciples, that a fruit ripens slowly but a day comes when it falls from the tree. Progress on the spiritual path is not at an even pace. We may 'ripen' at a particular pace, but liberation can suddenly occur at any moment. So, have faith and keep on at your journey.

Remembrance is the third component mentioned here. What are we supposed to remember? We are supposed to remember our spiritual practice. If our practice is to be aware of the breath, then we must remember to do this throughout the day, even when we are experiencing problems in our daily lives. If our practice is to stop all thoughts and remain in the present moment, then we must remember to do this during our waking hours.

21

Tīvra-saṁvegānām āsannaḥ

This is near for those with an intense desire for liberation.

Our liberation does not need to take much time, it can happen very quickly. It depends on the intensity of our desire for it. Desire is a very powerful tool of creation. What we desire deeply is what manifests in our lives. A desire that is pure and true, brings about a rapid transformation in our lives. Sometimes, a near-death experience can bring about a change in our focus and a longing for enlightenment. Imagine you are a person who has been diagnosed with COVID-19. Your best friend dies of the disease the same day you have tested positive for it. He lasts just four days in the hospital. Two days later, you are in hospital. The doctor tells you that you are on day 5 of the disease and from day 7, the virus becomes more virulent. Days 7 to 11 are critical for you. You are not sure whether you are living or dying, or whether you will ever see your family again. When you survive an experience like that, you realize that your body is mortal and you have a limited time with it on this planet. You can then choose to focus on what matters most to you, especially your enlightenment.

There are some very successful people who have turned spiritual and worked intensely toward their liberation. Their success has not satisfied them and left them with a feeling of emptiness. They come to the realization that material success does not leave one satisfied. Are these sensory pleasures all there is to life? Isn't there something more to life than this? These are some of the questions that arise in their mind. A poor person may believe that only material wealth is required for happiness. This is true to some extent when one is extremely poor and lacks the basics in life. But a successful person realizes that success and wealth do not bring happiness. Our problems do not go away, they may only become bigger. Patanjali explains at the end of the book why this happens. So, a successful person who has tasted the emptiness of success may then shift gears and focus on their enlightenment.

22

Mṛdu-madhyādhimātratvāt tato 'pi viśeṣaḥ

That also depends on whether the intensity is weak, moderate, or strong.

The intensity of your desire for enlightenment can be weak, moderate, or strong. If it is weak, it may take a few lifetimes to be enlightened. If the intensity is strong, it will happen in this lifetime.

Imagine you are baking a cake. If you keep getting up every 30 seconds and start doing something else, your cake will never get baked. It is the same with enlightenment. If you keep changing your attention to something else, then your enlightenment is going to take a very long time. Ultimately, it is a matter of focus. How focused are you on your goal? The more focused you are, the faster you will attain your goal. This is true of any goal, material or spiritual. The *Spanda Karikas* (33–37) explains this very well:

According to the desire abiding in the heart, God brings about the creation of what has been desired.

Since initially one's goal manifests unclearly. However, on constant attention of the mind on it, the object is made to manifest most clearly, through the continuous exercise of one's power.

So, in reality, remaining focussed on the desire is the manner by which desired objects are manifested. Therefore, by seizing that power, one is able to manifest a desire very quickly.

23

Īśvara-praṇidhānād vā

Or from service to God.

The path of service is very powerful. It can lead one rapidly to God. We place the needs of others above our own, which helps dissolve our ego. Patanjali discusses the path of service twice in the next chapter. Service to God is a part of the second limb of yoga—the *niyamas.*

Service to God is the same thing as service to life because God and life are the same. We serve by acting consciously from a state of awareness. Then, we will do what is required in that situation. When we act with awareness, we allow consciousness, or God, to manifest through us. We become aligned with life and our soul's higher purpose. We may end up changing what we do for a living, or we may remain in the same job but start performing it with a completely different attitude. When we serve God, we establish a connection with the Divine.

When you are able to surrender and connect to your deity, all fears disappear from your life. You know that God or Goddess will take care of you. Whenever you face a problem, you know it will be handled; God will take care of it. When you have this attitude, your health, wealth, and relationships improve. This realization that God takes care of us is open to everyone, not just those on the path of service. However, those serving God have a stronger connection with the Divine, so they come to this realisation faster. Ramana Maharshi used to say that when we board a train, we can put our bag down. We do not need to unnecessarily strain ourselves by continuously carrying it. The train will take us and our bag to the destination. In the same way, God always takes care of us and our needs. We do not need to unnecessarily strain ourselves by constantly worrying about our problems.

24

Kleśa-karma-vipākāśayair aparāmṛṣṭaḥ puruṣa-viśeṣa Īśvaraḥ

God is a special Soul, untouched by afflictions, actions, fruits of actions and the karmic process.

God is untouched by suffering of any kind, or by the karmic process. Patanjali explains the karmic process later but he mentions the key ingredients here—actions, consequences of actions, and fruits of previous actions that are stored until they ripen into an experience. The word *aśaya* has been translated here as the karmic process but it literally means, 'stock or fruits of past actions that are stored until they ripen into an experience.'

Many commentators of this text have used this Sutra to explain that Patanjali believes in a dualistic philosophy. That God is a special soul, separate from the rest of us, who are ordinary souls. We suffer, whereas God does not. We are bound by the karmic process whereas God is free of it. However, Patanjali is using dualistic language here because our present experience of life is dualistic. We experience life in a way that feels we are separate from God. The actual truth is different. Patanjali turns this philosophy on its head in the next chapter when he goes deeper into ultimate reality.

25

Tatra niratiśāyaṁ sarvajña-bījam

In God, is the source of omniscience that is unsurpassed.

Omniscience literally means to know everything. Its meaning here is broader. God is the source of all knowledge, wisdom, and intelligence. God's knowledge, wisdom, and intelligence are unsurpassed. Even the sharpest human mind contains a fraction of the intelligence that God has. The moon does not have any light of its own. It only reflects the light from the sun, which is why we are able to see it. The human mind is somewhat similar. Whatever wisdom or intelligence it contains, come from God, or from our soul, which is the part of God that is within us. The mind's wisdom and intelligence are insignificant when compared to the intelligence of God. That is why we are advised in moments of great difficulty, to still the mind and go within. When we still the noise of the mind, we are able to access the wisdom of the soul. We get ideas for solutions to some of our largest problems. So, when you are in difficulty, go to the source of wisdom and intelligence—go to God. You will find all the solutions there.

Sometimes, life takes a little time to work things out. Werner Erhard put it accurately when he said, 'Life resolves itself in the process of life itself.' One has to be patient and trust the process of life, even in our darkest moments. Life has a way of turning things around very fast.

26

Pūrveṣām api guruḥ kālenānavacchedāt

Unbound by time, God is the Guru even for those who came before.

God is the eternal master as God is not bound by time. God is the Guru not only for those who came before us, but also for those who will come after us.

27

Tasya vācakaḥ praṇavaḥ

The sound expressing him is AUM.

AUM is a mantra. It is a very powerful mantra. Mantras are sacred sounds that do not usually mean anything but have the power to liberate us. The sound that expresses God is AUM. The sound AUM, or a variation of it, is found in all major religions. In Hinduism and Buddhism, over time, the sound AUM has been modified to OM. In Christianity, the word 'Amen' and in Islam the word, 'Amin', is used at the end of prayers.

28

Taj-japas tad-artha-bhāvanam

Continuous recitation of it will manifest its meaning.

Reciting AUM will manifest it's meaning. This means that God will manifest within us, and we will be liberated.

There are other mantras used for liberation. Most mantras should be practiced under the guidance of a Guru. Mantras are very powerful sounds and if they are practiced incorrectly, they can even harm one. However, AUM is perfectly safe to chant. Patanjali has given us a mantra that is safe for everyone to practice.

How does one recite AUM? The correct way to pronounce it is AUM, not OM. There are only three sounds we can make without moving our tongue. They are A, U and M. If we open our mouth and make a sound, it will be 'aaa'. If we start closing our mouth, then the 'a' sound will become 'uuu', when the mouth is semi closed. Finally, when the mouth is fully closed, the 'u' sound becomes 'mmm.' Make the AUM sound while exhaling. Breathe in and while breathing out, make the sound 'aaa'. Then start closing the mouth. Automatically the 'aaa' sound will become 'uuu' and finally, 'mmm'. Then, breathe in and while exhaling, repeat this process.

29

Tataḥ pratyak-cetanādhigamo 'py antarāyābhāvaś ca

From this practice, consciousness turns inwards, and all obstacles are destroyed as well.

Normally, our mind constantly goes outwards toward the external world. When we chant AUM, the mind starts becoming still and our attention goes inwards toward the Self. The obstacles that are destroyed are mentioned in the next Sutra.

30

Vyādhi-styāna-saṁśaya-pramādālasyāvirati-bhrānti-darśanālabdha-bhūmikatvānavasthitatvāni citta-vikeṣepās te 'ntarāyāḥ

Disease, dullness, doubt, carelessness, laziness, intemperance, false perception, lack of depth in meditation, and unsteadiness. These distractions of the mind are the obstacles.

What are the obstacles in our spiritual journey? Patanjali lists the important ones here. Disease or illness prevents us from continuing our spiritual journey. We have to focus on regaining our health before we can restart our practices. Dullness refers to a lack of intelligence. This causes us to make incorrect decisions. Doubt results in a lack of commitment. We are not sure whether the spiritual path we have chosen is the correct one. Sometimes there is also self-doubt. We doubt our own ability to progress on the spiritual path. Carelessness causes us to perform our practices incorrectly, which results in slow progress. Laziness means we are not persevering in our practices and do not perform them regularly. Intemperance means a lack of moderation or restraint. It refers to a person who is overindulgent, usually with alcohol but it could also be with other sensory pleasures. Such people are more focused on experiencing sensory pleasures, than on their spiritual journey. False perception means we perceive things incorrectly and make incorrect decisions, which affects our spiritual progress. Lack of depth in meditation, results in slow progress and one does not gain the rewards of meditation. Finally, unsteadiness means that a person is not firmly committed to a path. They are easily distracted and think of other things.

All of these are distractions of the mind, and they are the obstacles to our spiritual progress.

31

**Duḥkha-daurmanasyāṅgam-ejayatva-śvāsa-
praśvāsā vikṣepa-saha-bhuvaḥ**

Suffering, despair, trembling of the body, and irregular breathing. These arise along with the distractions.

There is a saying that most diseases come from the mind. It is what Patanjali is implying. The distractions of the mind mentioned in the previous Sutra cause suffering, despair, and health problems. Today, trembling of the body is a sign of Parkinson's disease. Parkinson's is a nervous system disorder caused by certain nerve cells in the brain breaking down or dying. Irregular breathing can be a sign of asthma or hypertension The distraction of the mind causes all these health problems.

A distracted or uncontrolled mind is the cause of suffering and despair. When things go wrong, our mind is quick to judge these events and label them as 'wrong' or 'bad.' An event of its own, no matter how terrible, does not cause suffering. It is our thought about it that causes pain and anguish. The Greek philosopher Epictetus said, 'We are disturbed not by what happens to us, but by our thoughts about what happened.' Remove that thought and there is no suffering. Epictetus has been an inspiration to people for centuries, including American prisoners of war in Vietnam. One of them, James Stockdale, credits Epictetus for helping him endure the torture he was subjected to. He was put in leg irons, then he remembered that Epictetus had a disabled leg. Epictetus said, 'Sickness is a hindrance to your body, but not to your ability to choose unless that is your choice. Lameness is a hindrance to your leg, but not to your ability to choose.' He further said that you could say this about everything that happens to you, and you will understand that such obstacles are a hindrance to something else, but not to you.

32

Tat-pratiṣedhārtham eka-tattvābhyāsaḥ

For preventing them, continuously practice on the one true element.

To prevent suffering, despair, and health problems, such as trembling of the body and irregular breath, continuously chant the mantra AUM. AUM is the one true element referred to in this sutra. Chanting of AUM not only destroys all the obstacles mentioned in sutra 30, but it also destroys the suffering and health problems mentioned in the previous sutra.

How does this happen? Chanting of AUM raises our consciousness and stills the mind. Suffering and the health problems mentioned above are caused by a disturbed mind. When the mind is calm, suffering or health problems do not arise. Today, modern medicine has no cure for certain chronic health ailments, such as diabetes, hypertension, and asthma. At best, medicines help to control these illnesses. However, practices of yoga greatly help in the treatment of these illnesses and in many cases, even cure the patient completely. This is because the source of these illnesses is an agitated mind. Yoga gets to the root cause and treats these illnesses at the source. Once the mind becomes peaceful, these illnesses disappear or reduce greatly.

33

Maitrī-karuṇā-muditopekṣaṇāṁ
sukha-duḥkha-puṇyāpuṇya-viṣayāṇāṁ
bhāvanātaś citta-prasādanam

From being friendly toward the happy, compassionate toward the suffering, joyful to the virtuous and disregarding toward the wicked, brings about calmness of mind.

Patanjali now gives us some practical and useful advice, on how to live peacefully in this world. He divides people into four basic categories. We will encounter a variety of people in our life. They will come from different nationalities, religions, and races and have different personalities. However, they will all fit into one of the four categories: they will either be happy, be suffering, be virtuous, or be wicked. Patanjali tells us how to be with each of these types of people, to have a calm mind. This is important because we are usually disturbed by people. We are sometimes disturbed by the events in our life, but usually those events are caused by people. So how do we interact with these four types of people?

Being friendly toward happy people and joyful toward the virtuous, is relatively easy. These two types of people do not bring us pain, they bring us happiness. It is important to show compassion toward the suffering or the unhappy. The Sanskrit word for compassion is *karuṇā*. Compassion or *karuṇā*, is a wonderful quality to have. People with compassion have certainly evolved to a great degree. There are some who believe that Patanjali focuses mainly on detachment. This is only partly correct. Patanjali says it is important to be detached toward sensory objects. Without this detachment, it will be very difficult to still the mind. But he does not say that one should be detached in all moments of one's life. To be detached toward someone who is suffering, is cruel. We have to show compassion and help the suffering.

The fourth category of people, the wicked, is the most important. They are the ones who disturb us. Wicked here means people who are downright evil and also those who may not be evil but may have done something to hurt us. The word *upekṣa* has been translated here as disregarding. Its literal meaning is to overlook, disregard, or be indifferent. *Upekṣa* means we should overlook, disregard, or be indifferent to the faults of the wicked and accept them for who they are. This does not mean we should agree with what they have done or not try and change it but that we should accept them for the type of person they are. When we are able to do this, we no longer keep thinking about the evil things that have been done to us and our mind is at peace. To disregard or overlook other's faults and to forgive, is a wonderful thing. When we do not forgive others and store hatred within us, it is we who get affected. If you keep rubbish within you, it is your body that will rot. Buddha said something similar. He said: "He abused me, he beat me, he defeated me, he robbed me—in those who harbour such thoughts, hatred will never cease. He abused me, he beat me, he defeated me, he robbed me—in those who do not harbor such thoughts, hatred will cease. For hatred does not cease by hatred at any time; hatred ceases by love—this is an eternal law".

34

Pracchardana-vidhāraṇābhyāṁ vā prāṇasya

Or, by exhalation and retention of the breath.

In the next few sutras, Patanjali gives us some more ways to reach the state of Samadhi. The breath is in some way linked to the mind. What happens to the breath affects the mind. When the breath slows down, so does the mind. When the breath stops, the mind also becomes still. By exhaling and then holding the breath, the activity of the mind slows down. Of course, we cannot keep holding our breath, otherwise we would not survive. We need to breathe in again and then repeat this process—exhale and then retain the breath. When we achieve some proficiency in this practice, a time will come when the mind becomes still, and we enter the state of Samadhi.

The breath has an immediate effect on the body and mind. If we are tensed or nervous about something, one of the easiest ways to relax is to take a deep long breath; to breathe in and out deeply and slowly. It immediately has a calming effect on the mind. Some sportsmen use this method to calm themselves before a major sporting event.

The breath also has an effect on our life span. Animals, such as dogs and rabbits, breathe faster than humans (more breaths per minute) and have a shorter life span. Others, such as tortoises, breathe slower than humans and have a longer life span.

35

Viṣayavatī vā pravṛttir utpannā manasaḥ sthiti-nibandhanī

Or, this state arises, through steadiness in fixing the mind on an object of sense.

Meditation on an object of sense could be looking at something, like a picture of your favorite deity, or listening to something, like the sound of your breath. When you are able to fix your mind steadily on this object, without a break in your concentration, then the state of Samadhi arises within you.

Patanjali goes into greater detail about the various stages of meditation in Chapters Two and Three. Over here, he summarizes the main point—that you are able to focus on an object of sense steadily.

36

Viśokā vā jyotiṣmatī

Or, by focusing on the luminous Self within, that is untouched by sorrow.

Focussing on the *Self* is a very important practice. It has been given as a means for liberation by several masters, over the centuries. The Self is our soul. It is the witness within us that observes all the events of our life. That is why we are sometimes advised, "Be a witness." Being a witness means being aware. In a state of awareness, some of our attention is directed back toward the Self. Normally, we are lost in our thoughts, or all our attention is directed outwards. When we direct some of our attention inwards, to the Self, we become Self-aware. This is simply living in the present moment.

What exactly is the Self? The Self is consciousness. As spiritual sutras go, there are two sutras that are given more importance—this text, the *Yoga Sutras* of Patanjali, and the *Shiva Sutras.* There is an interesting story on how the *Shiva Sutras* was revealed. The legends say that Lord Shiva appeared to the sage Vasugupta in a dream and asked him to go to a particular stone near a stream. Vasugupta went there the next day and on touching the stone, the stone turned over, and on its face were inscribed the *Shiva Sutras.* The first sutra in the *Shiva Sutras* states, "*The Self is Consciousness.*"

Vasugupta wrote another book called, *The Spanda Karikas.* One of the fundamental life questions he asks in *The Spanda Karikas* is—What gives life to the body? And what is responsible for its creation, maintenance, and destruction? The answer is consciousness. He said, only by being in constant contact with consciousness, can there be existence.

The enlightened master, Sri Ramakrishna also said that everything is made up of consciousness: "The Divine Mother revealed to me in the Kali temple that it was she who had become everything. She showed me that everything was full of Consciousness. The image was Consciousness, the water was Consciousness, the altar was Consciousness, the water vessels were Consciousness, the doorsills were Consciousness, the marble floor was Consciousness—all was Consciousness."

The master who probably explained it best was Ramana Maharshi. He said that while the phenomena we see in the external world may be interesting, what we do not realize is that there is only one unlimited force that is responsible for all that we see and the act of seeing them. He said we should direct our attention inward on *That* (the Self), which sees all things and is responsible for everything, rather than the changing phenomena of the external world. He further said that an actor remains aware that he is an actor, no matter what part he plays. In the same way, we should not confuse ourselves with our body and should have a firm awareness of being the Self.

37

Vīta-rāga-viṣayaṁ vā cittam

Or, when the mind is free from attachment to any sense object.

Patanjali has mentioned detachment from sense objects earlier, in sutras 12 and 15. He is repeating it as it is important. If we are attached to objects of sense, it becomes difficult to still the mind. If we are constantly thinking of acquiring or experiencing food, money, sex, clothes, cars, houses, mobiles, etc., then the activities of the mind will not subside.

Sense objects are enjoyed by the body. When we constantly crave sense objects, we are deeply identified with the body. When we become free of attachment to sense objects, we are no longer identified with the body but with the Self. We are then able to enter the state of Samadhi.

38

Svapna-nidrā-jñānālambanaṁ vā

Or, knowing that which supports the state of dreaming and deep sleep.

What supports the dream state and the state of deep sleep? Consciousness supports both these states. This may be a little hard to believe as there is no awareness or consciousness in the state of deep sleep. However, consciousness is the basic life-giving force which supports everything.

The Sutra says that if we know consciousness (that which supports these two states), then we can reach Samadhi. Knowing consciousness means that we are in a state of consciousness or awareness, most of the time. In a conscious state, our mind is still, and we can attain Samadhi.

39

Yathābhimata-dhyānād vā

Or, by meditating on whatever is dear to one.

When we meditate on an object, it should be something that is dear to us, so that it holds our attention for a long period of time. If we meditate on something that means nothing to us, our mind will be easily distracted, and we will not be able to focus on it for long. It is for this reason that we are given complete freedom to choose whatever we wish to meditate on.

At a time when India's population was only 30 million, there were probably about 30 million Gods and Goddesses that were worshipped. Later, when the invaders came into the country, they could not understand how there could be such a multiplicity of divine forms that were worshipped. The Divine was worshipped in multiple forms for a very good reason. All created forms are a part of the Divine. We can use any aspect of creation as a gateway to enter the Divine. If we found a rock, a tree, or a mountain sacred, we were free to worship them and use them as a gateway to reach God. That was the amazing thing about the spiritual system that was prevalent in this country—the freedom given to an individual to decide what was sacred to them, and to use that for their liberation. From this freedom of worship arose tolerance. When you allowed someone to worship the Divine in whichever form they chose, then you were no longer forcing your God, or your belief system onto them. This was the basis of the tolerance found in India.

40

Paramāṇu-parama-mahattvānto 'sya vaśīkāraḥ

This yogi's mastery extends from the smallest particle to the end of the largest one.

Yoga teaches us that all matter is made up of just five elements—earth, water, fire, air, and space. Everything is just a combination of these five elements, from the smallest particle to the largest one. The sutra starts by saying, "*This yogi's mastery*". This is a reference to someone who has attained Samadhi. The past few sutras have given us a few methods for attaining Samadhi. The yogi who has attained Samadhi gains mastery over the five elements. Since everything, from the smallest particle to the end of the largest one, is only made of these five elements, the yogi becomes a master of all the particles in this world.

Chapter Three examines in detail, the powers gained by a yogi who has attained Samadhi and the dangers they present.

41

Kṣīṇa-vṛtter abhijātasyeva maṇer grahītṛ-grahaṇa-grāhyeṣu tat-stha-tad-añjanatā samāpattiḥ

Samapatti is the state when the activities of the mind have subsided and the mind becomes similar to a pure crystal, which reflects the colours of any object placed near it. In this state, the perceiver, the perceived object, and the perceiving of it, appear one.

Patanjali is now finally going to explain what Samadhi is. First, he explains the state of Samapatti. Samapatti occurs just before Samadhi and can even be explained as the beginning of Samadhi.

When you are meditating on an object, say for example, a picture of your favorite deity, a stage comes when the mind becomes fairly still. Its activities have subsided, and it becomes pure like a crystal. If you place an object near a crystal, it reflects the colour of that object. Similarly, the mind in this state, reflects the object. The object (in this case the picture of the deity), the meditator, and the means of perceiving the object, appear one.

42

Tatra śabdārtha-jñāna-vikalpaiḥ saṁkīrṇā savitarkā-samāpattiḥ

In that state, the distinction between the sound (perceiver), the object, and the knowing of it, is all mixed up. This is Savitarka Samapatti.

In that state, there is no distinction between the meditator, the object being meditated on, and the knowing of it. It is all mixed up, and everything appears one. Normally, when we meditate, we are aware of the distinction between ourselves and the object we are meditating on. We are also aware of the way we are perceiving an object. If we are meditating on a picture of our deity, we are aware of ourselves, and the picture, and we are using our eyesight to meditate on the picture. In the advanced state of Samapatti, the distinction between the three is gone and it all appears as one.

Patanjali calls this state, Savitarka Samapatti.

43

Smṛti-pariśuddhau svarūpa-śūnyevārtha -mātra-nirbhāsā nirvitarkā

When the memory is cleansed, it seems like one's own form is non-existent, and the object only appears. This is Nirvitarka (Samadhi).

The next stage is when our memory is cleansed, and it seems that our own form is non-existent. In this state, only the object appears. This is *Nirvitarka Samadhi*. Patanjali defines Samadhi in this sutra. He explains it once more, in the third sutra of Chapter Three, and he says the same thing there.

Patanjali is using a few technical words here, but don't let that overwhelm you. The meanings of these words are fairly simple. Samapatti is the state where the distinction between the meditator, the object being meditated on, and the means of perception, is mixed up, and they all appear as one. In Samadhi, our own form appears to be non-existent and only the object appears.

What does Savitarka and Nirvitarka mean? *Sa* is a prefix that means 'with' and *Nir* is a prefix that means 'without.' Savitarka means, 'with vitarka' and Nirvitarka means, 'without vitarka.' Vitarka means doubt, uncertainty, deliberation, and reflection. Savitarka literally means 'with doubt', and Nirvitarka means, 'without doubt.' However, given what Patanjali has said in this sutra, he is using vitarka to mean 'memory.' Savitarka, 'with memory', means there is some memory of one's form, even though the Meditator and the object being meditated on, appear as one. Nirvitarka, 'without memory,' of one's form, and only the object appears.

44

Etayaiva savicārā nirvicārā ca sūkṣma-viṣayā vyākhyātā

By the same way, Savicara and Nirvicara, which are practiced on subtle objects, are explained.

Vicara has the same meaning as vitarka. They both mean doubt, deliberation, or reflection. In the context used by Patanjali, it means memory. Savicara and Nirvicara have the same meaning as Savitarka and Nirvitarka, respectively. Savicara and Nirvicara are used when meditation is practiced on subtle objects. For example, the sound of our breath is subtle. Listening to the sound of one's breath is a meditation on a subtle object. If we attained Samadhi by meditating on a subtle object, it would be called Nirvicara Samadhi.

45

Sūkṣma-viṣayatvaṁ cāliṅga-paryavasānam

And the subtleness of the object being meditated on extends up to the imperceptible.

The subtleness of the object being meditated on can reach a point where it is no longer perceptible. The following example from the *Vigyan Bhairava Tantra* (Verse 39), will make this clear:

O Goddess, chant AUM, etc., slowly. Concentrate on the void at the end of the protracted sound. Then with the supreme energy of the Void, one goes to the Void.

One practices the above meditation by chanting AUM slowly. Focus on the end of the sound. You will first hear the sound gradually diminishing and ending. Then, you will feel its vibration for a few seconds more. Finally, there will be silence, which is the Void referred to in meditation. So, the practice starts with sound, then goes to the vibration of the sound, and finally to silence. At each stage, it gets subtler and subtler till finally, there is nothing—only the Void.

46

Tā eva sabījaḥ samādhiḥ

These are all in fact, Samadhi with seed (Sabija).

Sabija is made up of two words—*Sa* which means 'with', and *bija* with means 'seed.' *Sabija* means, 'with seed.' The Samadhi's discussed in the previous few sutras are all Samadhi's with seed. The seed referred to, is the seed of our rebirth. While this seed is still in existence, we will be reborn. To attain final liberation, this seed needs to be destroyed. Patanjali explains in the following sutras what this seed exactly is and how it is destroyed.

47

Nirvicāra-vaiśāradye 'dhyātma-prasādaḥ

With expertise in Nirvicara, the Supreme Self shines.

When we attain the state of Nirvicara Samadhi, our Supreme Self, or our soul, shines. We do not experience our *Self* when our mind is active. In the state of Nirvicara Samadhi, the mind has fallen silent; therefore, we experience our Supreme Self in all its dimensions.

48

ṛtam-bharā tatra prajñā

That state carries divine truth, which is wisdom.

The state of Nirvicara Samadhi is divine, where the individual is absent. That state carries divine truth, which is wisdom. The word *prajñā* (pronounced *prug-yaa*), has been translated here as wisdom. It also means intelligence and knowledge. All three meanings apply here. Samadhi is a state of high consciousness. Consciousness has a certain intelligence. This is the intelligence of the Creator. In the state of Samadhi, we access that wisdom and intelligence. Intelligence is different from intellect. Our intellect has a certain amount of intelligence, but it is extremely limited compared to Divine intelligence.

It is possible to access some of this Divine wisdom on a daily basis. When we face a problem, usually our mind reacts to it. Instead, keep the mind quiet and you will find a response coming from within you. This response is from your soul. It is the intelligence of the Creator and will show us the best way forward.

49

Śrutānumāna-prajñābhyām anya-viṣayā viśeṣārthatvāt

This wisdom because of its extraordinary sense, belongs to a different realm from the wisdom heard from scriptures, or from inference.

Divine wisdom has extraordinary sense. It belongs to a different level compared to wisdom heard from scriptures, or from inference. It is for this reason we seek to remember every word spoken by a master, or an enlightened saint. When we listen to scriptures or infer something, we are still routing everything through our mind. In Samadhi there is a direct connection to the Source, and it is in this state that we receive true wisdom.

Sometimes a master can help us reach Samadhi through their grace. Paul Brunton was one of the twentieth century's great spiritual explorers. He came to India and lived amongst yogis, mystics, and Gurus, trying to find one, who would give him peace and tranquillity. His search ended with Ramana Maharshi. He chronicled his journey in his book titled *A Search In Secret India.* He spent a considerable amount of time in Ramana Maharshi's ashram in South India. Once, shortly before he left, he joined the evening meditation practice late. The Maharshi was seated at the head of the hall. To his surprise he found when he started his meditation, he went deep very quickly. Then suddenly, thoughts got extinguished and he found consciousness working unhindered. He remained in that state for two hours and received several insights. Amongst them:

A person who has met his real Self will never again hate someone else.

We should place our worldly troubles and burdens, into the beautiful care of our Self, and it will not fail us.

We may delve deep into ancient manuscripts, but we will find no higher truth than that our very Self is divine.

50

Taj-jaḥ saṁskāro 'nya-saṁskāra-pratibandhī

The impression produced by that state, destroys all other impressions.

There is a word used in this sutra, *Saṁskāra* (pronounced Sanskaara), that is repeated throughout the text and has been translated here as impressions. It is an important word to understand. *Saṁskāras* are basically a storehouse of karma. It is the stock, or the fruits of our past actions, that are stored until they ripen into existence. These actions may have been done in this lifetime, or in a previous form of existence. This storehouse of karma is stored in the mind in the form of impressions.

While these impressions, or stock of karma exists, the seed of our future births will always be there. We are reborn till our stock of karma lasts. Once it is exhausted or destroyed, then there is no possibility of our rebirth, and we can achieve liberation.

In the state of Nirvicara Samadhi, there is an impression (*Saṁskāra*) produced that destroys all our existing impressions. This new impression destroys our entire storehouse of karma.

51

Tasyāpi nirodhe sarva-nirodhān nirbījaḥ samādhiḥ

On the destruction of even that impression, all impressions are destroyed, and one attains Nirbija (seedless) Samadhi.

Once this new impression destroys all existing impressions, it also gets destroyed and we reach a state of Samadhi where there are no impressions left. This Samadhi is called *Nirbija*, which literally means, "without seed", or seedless. In Nirbija Samadhi, there is no stock of karma left and therefore no seed for rebirth, which is why it is called seedless Samadhi.

Our storehouse of karma is responsible for our sense of individuality. We exist as a separate individual with our own personality because we have a stock of karma. When our karma gets destroyed, our individual self dissolves, and we merge with the Divine and attain liberation.

So, is Nirbija Samadhi a state of liberation? Well, almost. Patanjali does not say anything more here because there is one more step to be taken for liberation, which he explains in Chapters Three and Four.

CHAPTER TWO

SĀDHANA PĀDA

SPIRITUAL PRACTICE

In this chapter, Patanjali goes into greater detail on the spiritual practices to be performed, for attaining Samadhi and liberation. The chapter could be divided into two equal halves, with the second half devoted to the eight limbs of yoga.

1

Tapaḥ-svādhyāyeśvara-praṇidhānāni kriyā-yogaḥ

Austerities, study of sacred scriptures and service to God, constitute Kriya Yoga.

Patanjali starts with Kriya Yoga. Kriya Yoga is the path of selfless action and has three components—practice of austerities, study of sacred scriptures and service to God. Each of these three components are part of the second limb of yoga and are described again, at the end of this chapter.

Austerities are practices that purify and energise the body. They are very helpful for people leading an active life, especially a life of service.

Study of sacred scriptures ensures that we are on the path to liberation. These scriptures guide us and put us on the right path. Patanjali had mentioned in sutra 1.7 that authoritative scriptures are one source of forming right beliefs. He underlines their importance again for Kriya Yoga.

Service to God by itself, is sufficient for our liberation. Patanjali considers it so important that he mentions it three times in this text.

Today, Kriya Yoga means something completely different. It now refers to meditation practices performed to reach enlightenment. Kriya literally means action, activity, work. The word *praṇidhānā* given in this sutra, is sometimes translated as devotion. However, *praṇidhānā* means service, not devotion. Kriya Yoga is the path of selfless action, not the path of worship. The path of devotion is a beautiful path but it is not what Patanjali is referring to here. Patanjali is referring to the path of action, where one works without being attached to rewards. Lord Krishna called this Karma Yoga in the *Bhagavad Gita*. Kriya and Karma, are two Sanskrit words that both mean action. The Kriya Yoga mentioned here is the same as the Karma Yoga described in the *Bhagavad Gita*. In the *Bhagavad Gita* (2.47–48), Karma Yoga is explained in the following way:

You have a right only to your work, not at any time on its rewards. Do not let the rewards be the motive for your actions and neither become attached to inaction.

Give up selfish desires while performing actions, O Arjuna. This is being established in yoga. Be the same in success and in failure. This equanimity is called yoga.

In this path, ones uses action, or one's work as a means for liberation. You can serve Life through your work. Lord Krishna explains that you have a right to your work, not to its rewards. You may become very successful in your work and earn lots of money. However, you should become a trustee or steward of the wealth you have earned. You should share the wealth with those who need it. For example, in a forest you will find that monkeys only consume the amount of food that they need. If a monkey gathered most of the fruit and hoarded it, and there were some monkeys who starved for lack of food, we would think there was something wrong with that monkey. However, human beings who display this behaviour are called successful. Lord Krishna is saying that we should not claim ownership for the rewards of our work. We should also not let the rewards be the motive for our actions.

In verse 2.48, Lord Krishna states that we should give up selfish desires while performing actions. Patanjali explains the Law of Karma in this chapter and Chapter Four. As we will learn later, it is the motive behind our actions that cause Karma. When are actions are not based on selfish desires, or when we choose to serve God, then the karmic process ceases to entangle us.

The importance of serving God, is also emphasised in other traditions. Neale Donald Walsch, in his bestselling book, *Tomorrow's God*, asks God a fundamental question about life—How do we function within this illusory world and still find peace, harmony and happiness? What is the secret formula? God gives the answer in one word—service. He explains, service to God means service to Life because they are the same thing. When you serve Life, Life serves you because you and Life are one. However, you cannot serve Life first if you think that you individually lack something. You will then end up serving your needs. You serve Life when the needs of others become more important than your own needs When you understand that you and Life are one, you will realize that serving Life is actually serving your Self. This is a major step toward becoming a Master.

Service to God does not necessarily mean one gives up one's profession and becomes a social worker. We can serve others through our existing profession. It requires a change in our attitude and a commitment to help and serve others. One also has to work consciously. It means living fully in the present moment and acting with awareness. One does not have to change what one is doing but *how* one is doing things. One gives full attention to this moment. A person can be a doctor, engineer, businessman, sportsman, or in any other profession. When you act from present moment awareness, you allow consciousness to flow through you into what you are doing. God is consciousness. When you act with consciousness, the energy of God flows into whatever you are doing. That is when you become creative and have the maximum impact in this world through what you are doing. When you act with awareness, your actions always serve life, irrespective of what profession you are in. On the other hand, you may have great intentions and do social work, but you need to be careful that the ego does not get into what you are doing. With ego, inevitably there is suffering, even with the best intentions.

2

**Samādhi-bhāvanārthaḥ
kleśa-tanū-karaṇārthaś ca**

Kriya Yoga is practiced for minimizing the afflictions and for bringing about Samadhi.

An affliction is something that causes suffering. Patanjali discusses the afflictions in greater detail in the next few sutras. Kriya Yoga reduces the causes of suffering in our lives (the afflictions) and brings about Samadhi.

3

Avidyāsmitā-rāga-dveṣābhiniveśāḥ kleśāḥ

The afflictions are: ignorance, egoism, attraction, aversion, and tenacity of mundane existence.

There are five afflictions listed by Patanjali. Each of them is discussed in greater detail.

4

Avidyā kṣetram uttareṣāṁ prasupta-tanu-vicchinnodārāṇām

Ignorance is the source of the subsequent afflictions, whether they are dormant, weak, intermittent, or strong.

Ignorance is the main affliction. All other afflictions arise from ignorance. The afflictions fall into four categories—they may be dormant and may not have arisen; they may be weak; they may be intermittent, that is they may come and go; finally, they may be strong. It does not matter which category they belong to, but all the subsequent four afflictions come from ignorance.

5

Anityāśuci-duḥkhānātmasu nitya-śuci-sukhātma-khyātir avidyā

Ignorance is to perceive the transient as eternal, the impure as pure, pain as pleasure, and the non-self as the Self.

Ignorance is not just the cause of our suffering, it is also the cause of our bondage. As Patanjali makes clear later in this chapter, the removal of ignorance leads to our liberation.

Ignorance is divided into four parts. It is the last one, perceiving the non-self as the Self, which is the most important. All the other three are connected to it in some way. The first mistake we make is to believe the transient is eternal. We seek outward pleasures, not realising that these are transient and will pass away. The fact that we seek pleasures and try and avoid pain is one of the causes of our suffering.. Whatever we are seeking in this world, is transient and is not permanent. One of the most beautiful Upanishads, is the *Katha Upanishad*. It is a dialogue between Nachiketas, a young boy who is seeking the truth, and Yama, the God of Death. One of the pieces of advice Yama gives him, is not to seek the eternal in things that pass away. He says:

The ignorant go after outward pleasures and they fall into the trap of vast encompassing death. But the wise have a correct understanding of liberation and do not seek the eternal here, in things that pass away.

The second part of our ignorance is that we sometimes perceive created matter to be pure. However, whatever is created is not pure, only the Self, the Creator is pure. This is because created matter is subject to decay, but the Creator is imperishable.

Thirdly, Patanjali says that what we consider to be pleasure is actually pain. Pleasures of the body are nothing in comparison to pleasures of the soul. The joy and bliss of the Self is infinitely more pleasurably than pleasures of the body. What we consider to be pleasure, is actually pain when you compare it to the joy of the soul.

Finally, ignorance means we confuse the non–self for the Self. The second affliction, egoism arises from this. We mistake the body to be our real Self. This is explained in the next sutra.

6

Dṛg-darśana-śaktyor ekātmatevāsmitā

Egoism is identifying with the creation of the Seer—the instrument of experiencing (body and mind).

Egoism is our sense of individuality. It is when we identify with the instrument used by the Self to experience life, which is the body and mind. As explained earlier, Patanjali uses the word *asmitā* for the ego, which literally means I-ness. He also uses the word, Seer, for the Self, which is an apt way to describe the Self. The Self is consciousness, and the Seer is a beautiful way to describe consciousness.

Take the example of air. Air is found everywhere. If you put air inside a jar and closed it and the air forgot it was air, and believed it was the jar, then that is similar to the egoism that we are experiencing. If you break the jar, then the air once again unites with air outside. Similarly, we are the Self, not the body. The body is a tool for the Self to experience life. But somewhere we have forgotten we are the Self, and started believing we are the body. To be liberated, we need to break our identification with the body and dissolve our individuality.

Once we are identified with the body, we become influenced by pleasure and pain, which are the next two afflictions. You can see how one affliction leads to another.

7

Sukhānuśayī rāgaḥ

Being influenced by pleasure, is attraction.

8

Duḥkhānuśayī dveṣaḥ

Being influenced by pain, is aversion.

When we are influenced, affected, or impacted by pleasure, it is called attraction. Similarly, when we are influenced, affected, or impacted by pain, it is aversion. In simple terms, attraction and aversion is liking and disliking. We like pleasure, we dislike pain. We enjoy certain activities, we dislike other activities. For example, we enjoy going to our favourite restaurant for a meal and we dislike going to the crematorium for someone's funeral. We enjoy going on vacation but may not enjoy going to work. These likes and dislikes arise from our ego and karmic impressions. It is because we have an ego, or a personality, that we have certain likes and dislikes toward what we are doing. One of the fastest ways to evolve is to stop liking and disliking and be aware and accepting.

A master simply does what is required. They have no sense of being the "doer." As Ramana Maharshi said, a sage may be accomplishing a great many things, but he or she knows the truth that they are doing nothing, and they are the silent witness in whose presence these activities are taking place. When you do not identify yourself with the body, or as the "doer", you have no attraction or aversion toward any activity, and you are not affected by pleasure or pain.

The *Shiva Sutras* explains this nicely. It says, for a master, *Pleasure and pain are considered to be something external* (3.33). It continues, *But one who is shrunk by delusion believes the self performs actions* (3.35).

9

Svarasa-vāhī viduṣo 'pi tathārūḍho 'bhiniveśaḥ

The tenacity of mundane existence flows by its own force. This is pervasive even amongst the wise.

There is a certain resistance to change. We are so used to living the way we are, that it takes effort to break the cycle and move to a higher plane of existence. Our mundane way of living has its own force. Sometimes, we are scared of radically changing the way we exist. This fear of the unknown keeps us from fully committing to the spiritual path. This happens even to the wise. There is a story in Swami Vivekananda's life that illustrates this, described in the book, *Sri Ramakrishna, and His Divine Play*:

Swami Vivekananda's original name was Narendranath Datta. The second time he met Ramakrishna was at the Dakshineswar Temple. When he went to his room, he found Ramakrishna sitting deep in meditation on his bed. When he saw Narendra (later to become Swami Vivekananda), he joyfully called out to him and asked him to sit at the end of the bed. He then touched Vivekananda's body with his foot. Vivekananda immediately had an extraordinary experience. He felt everything in the room, including the walls, whirling around, and receding. He also felt the entire universe and his self being devoured by a vast void. That frightened him and he thought he might die. He cried out, "Ah, what are you doing to me? Don't you know I have parents at home?" When Ramakrishna heard this, he laughed loudly. Then he touched Vivekananda's chest with his hand and said, "All right, let it stop now. It needn't be done all at once. It will happen in its own good time." To Vivekananda's amazement, that extraordinary vision disappeared as quickly as it had come. He returned to his normal state and saw objects in the room standing as before. After this, Swami Vivekananda resolved to know the cause of that experience and not let it overwhelm him again in the future. Similarly, if we choose to, we can overcome the tenacity of ordinary existence and move to a higher plane of existence.

10

Te pratiprasava-heyāḥ sūkṣmāḥ

If these afflictions are weak, they can be destroyed by returning to the original state.

If the afflictions are weak, they can be destroyed by returning to the original state. The original state is a state of full awareness. If the afflictions are weak, it means that a person is already in a high state of awareness. Their level of ignorance is low and their ego is almost non-existent. Such a person needs to remain in awareness, to fully destroy the afflictions.

11

Dhyāna-heyās tad-vṛttayaḥ

If they are in an active state, they can be destroyed through meditation.

If the afflictions are active and strong, then they can be destroyed through meditation. If your level of ignorance is high, your ego is big, you have strong likes and dislikes, and you have a tenacity for ordinary existence, then all of these can be destroyed through meditation.

12

**Kleśa-mūlaḥ karmāśayo
dṛṣṭādṛṣṭa-janma-vedanīyaḥ**

The storehouse of Karma has its root in these afflictions. The fruits of Karma (action) are experienced in the present and future lives.

In the next three sutras, Patanjali discusses Karma and how it works. Karma means action. Some of our actions have consequences. The fruits or consequences of our actions are stored as impressions until they ripen into experience. They will ripen into experience either in the present life, or in future lives.

There are three types of karma—*Sanchita, Prarabdha,* and *Agami. Sanchita* is your entire storehouse of karma. *Prarabdha* is the amount of karma taken from that storehouse, for you to exhaust in this lifetime. It is the karma given to you to finish in this lifetime. *Agami* is the new karma that you are building up through your actions in this lifetime. It may take several lifetimes to exhaust your entire storehouse of karma and at the same time you are building up more karma through your actions in the present and future lifetimes.

The storehouse of karma has its root in these afflictions. Not all of our actions build up karma. Some actions create new karma, and some actions exhaust existing karma. Patanjali explains in Chapter Four, why some of our actions create karma and how we can prevent that. But he is giving us a hint here. The root lies in these afflictions. The basic cause of the storehouse of karma, is these afflictions. When we have an ego, we have likes and dislikes. When we act from that ego, or from our likes and dislikes, then our actions have consequences and build karma. When we act from a state of awareness or act to serve life, then our actions do not build any new karma but exhaust existing karma. That is why the first two sutras of this chapter, give Kriya Yoga, the path of service as a way of bringing about Samadhi. Kriya Yoga today is called Karma Yoga, the path of selfless action. There is a lot more to be said on this subject, which is discussed by Patanjali in Chapter Four.

When you start on a spiritual path, you have taken a decision that you do not wish to wait several lifetimes to exhaust your karma. You wish to accelerate this process. When you reach a state of Samadhi, your storehouse of karma automatically gets destroyed. As was explained at the end of the last chapter, in the state of Samadhi, a new impression is created, which destroys all existing impressions (our storehouse of karma).

13

Sati mūle tad-vipāko jāty-āyur-bhogāḥ

As long as the root exists, the fruits of action result in birth as a particular kind, for a life span, and various experiences.

As long as the afflictions exist, the root cause of karma exists and there will be consequences to our actions. These consequences or fruits of action, result in our birth as a particular type of person, with a certain life span, and with a variety of experiences. When we are born, we come with a certain amount of information. This information is like our software. Our genetic code is part of this software. The information determines what kind of person we are, what abilities we have or do not have, and also what experiences we have. Some of the experiences we have in this lifetime are a consequence of actions we have committed in a past lifetime. Other experiences are a result of actions we have taken in this lifetime. What this means, is that our lives are in our hands and of our own making. We are not ruled by fate. Our actions determine our future, in this and future lifetimes. When we understand this, we no longer blame anyone else for the conditions of our life. If we have an accident or some mishap, we know we are responsible for it due to our past actions. We will cease to blame another person for the accident, or for anything else that goes wrong in our lives.

Can we be born in a lower form of existence as a punishment for our evil actions? If we are a human being in this lifetime, can we be born as an animal, an insect, or some other lower life form, due to our misdeeds in this lifetime? Lord Krishna in the Bhagavad Gita (2.40) says that no step is lost in this path. He is implying that we cannot go backward in our evolution and that once we take a human form, we only evolve from there on. In this sutra, there is a word used—*jāti*. *Jāti* means 'kind, class, race, species, caste.' It has been translated here as 'kind.' Some translators have translated *jāti* as 'species.' They believe we can change into a different species at birth as a consequence of our actions. However, that is not what Patanjali is saying, as he makes clear in Chapter Four. He uses *jāti* to mean the type or kind of person, we are born as.

14

Te hlāda-paritāpa-phalāḥ puṇyāpuṇya-hetutvāt

These experiences of pleasure and pain are consequences, caused by being virtuous or wicked.

We experience pleasure as a consequence of being virtuous and pain as a consequence of being wicked. What you do to others, you will one day experience. The reason for this is simple—you and the other are actually one. What you think you are doing to another, you are actually doing to yourself and will experience it in this or future lifetimes. What you do to others will be done to you. What you fail to do for others, will fail to be done for you. What you give, you receive. This in a nutshell, is one of the Laws of Karma. This is true of all our relationships and even our work. We sometimes enter into a relationship hoping to find joy and happiness there. The only joy we will find in a relationship is the joy we put in, whether it is with our children, spouse, or anyone else. This also holds true with our work. If we expect to receive something without putting anything in, we are only going to end up disappointing ourselves. Ultimately, we are the source of the joy we experience in our lives. The joy we give out is the joy we receive.

15

Pariṇāma-tāpa-saṁskāra-duḥkhair
guṇa-vṛtti-virodhāc ca duḥkham
eva sarvaṁ vivekinaḥ

To one of discrimination, everything is suffering in fact. This is due to the suffering that is latent in the impressions, the sorrow over changing circumstances and the inherent contradictions in the functioning of the qualities of nature.

If you are a keen observer of life, you will realize that the outside world is all suffering. Buddhism was later to say the same thing.

The first sermon Buddha gave after enlightenment, was at the Deer Park, outside Varanasi. In that sermon, he enumerated the Four Noble Truths. The First Noble Truth is, 'All existence is suffering.'

Patanjali gives us three ways in which suffering appears in our lives. The first is suffering that is latent in the impressions, or our storehouse of karma. In our present lifetime or in our past lives, we may have committed certain wicked actions. The consequences of those wicked actions are currently lying latent in our storehouse of karma, but sometime in the future, those consequences will appear in our life and cause suffering. Secondly, we may suffer due to changing conditions. Our life may be very pleasant and may be going well. Then, suddenly we lose our job or face a major financial loss. Or a close family member or friend may lose their life. Or, we may fall sick. There are many things that could go wrong in our lives. It is when our lives take a turn for the worse, that we suffer.

Thirdly, there are inherent contradictions in the functioning of the qualities of nature. The specific qualities of nature are explained three sutras later. The important point to understand is that nature (the outside world), functions with inherent contradictions. If you believe that the outside world could give you only pleasant experiences, then you will be sadly disappointed. The outside world does not function like that. Nature has inherent, built-in contradictions in it. Life is cyclical. It has a series of dualities in it—day and night, good and evil, pain and pleasure. We strive for pleasures and try and avoid pain and that is why we suffer. We cannot have one experience and not the other. Patanjali explained in sutra 5 of this chapter, that what we consider to be pleasure, is actually pain. Compared to the bliss of the soul, bodily pleasures feel like pain.

So, how should one handle change and the inherent contradictions of the world, so that we no longer suffer? The

Ashtavakra Gita (11.1), explains that change is an inherent part of life and we need to change our perception about this:

All things arise, experience change and pass away. This is their inherent nature. When you understand this, you remain unperturbed and free from pain. Through this peace in fact, you become still.

Whatever is created will experience change and pass away. Whether it is a pleasant or unpleasant situation, or a person we love or hate. Everything experiences changes and passes away. Our present life situation is temporary. It too will change. That is why Lord Krishna in the *Bhagavad Gita* (2.14), advises us to be patient:

Contact with the physical world brings pleasure and pain, heat and cold. But Arjuna, they are transient; they come and they go. Have patience, O son of Bharata.

Some may view this sutra to be overly negative. It isn't. Patanjali is just being factual. The actual cause of our suffering is internal, not external. The cause of our suffering is the five afflictions given earlier in this chapter. We experience suffering in our lives because we have not removed these afflictions. Once they are gone, life is just beautiful. When you find inner peace, your inner Self, then the outside world no longer troubles you. Life is meant to be joy, not suffering. If life was only endless suffering, then what would be the purpose of life? It would be better to end our life. No, life was meant to be bliss. Patanjali shows us how to end suffering and reach a state of bliss. The next few sutras discuss this further.

16

Heyaṁ duḥkham anāgatam

Suffering that is yet to come, can be avoided.

Suffering that has not yet arisen in our lives, can be avoided.

17

Draṣṭṛ-dṛśyayoḥ saṁyogo heya-hetuḥ

The union of the Seer and the Seen, causes avoidance of this suffering.

The way to avoid suffering is to be liberated. The 'Seen', is the individual human being. The 'Seer', is the Self, the soul, or God. The union of the Seer and the Seen, is the union of the individual with the Divine. This union is sometimes called Self-realization. We make our Divine Self real in our experience. This is the true meaning of yoga. Yoga means union. It is the union of the individual with the Divine.

Many masters have said the same thing—liberation is the end of our suffering. We suffer because of our ego. Egoism or 'I-ness', is one of the afflictions mentioned earlier. The larger the ego, the more the suffering. Conversely, the smaller the ego, the more joy we experience in our lives. It is not external circumstances that are the cause of our suffering, but our inner reaction to them. It is our ego that is judgemental and has strong likes and dislikes. A liberated person has found the bliss of their Divine Self. They no longer need anything from the external world, and the external world ceases to have any hold on them. Then, there is no further possibility of suffering.

Someone once asked Nisargadatta Maharaj, whether the search for our Self was worth the trouble. He replied, that without it everything was trouble. If we want to live sanely, creatively, and happily, we must search for who we truly are.

18

Prakāśa-kriyā-sthiti-sīlaṁ bhūtendriyātmakaṁ bhogāpavargārthaṁ dṛśyam

The Seen consists of the sense organs and elements, and has the nature of inertia, activity, and illumination. Its purpose is both, experiencing life and liberation of the soul.

When Patanjali uses the term 'Seen', he is either referring to the individual human body, or the physical world in general. The body consists of the sense organs and the elements. There are five primary elements. These are water, earth, fire, air, and space. All physical matter is made up of these five elements in different proportions. Essentially, the physical world is a play of five elements. The human body is approximately 72% water. The ancient sages of India realized the impact the moon had on the human system. During a full moon and new moon night, the ocean tides rise. As our bodies are 72% water, there is a natural upsurge of energy in the human system, during these two days. These are very auspicious days for our spiritual practice. There are many people through the centuries, who were enlightened either on a full moon day, or a new moon day. Buddha was enlightened on a full moon day in the month of May.

Nature has three basic qualities, that are found in all physical matter: *Tamas*, which is lethargy or inertia, *Rajas* which is activity or dynamism, and *Sattva* which is balance or illumination. The quality of food we eat can affect us as human beings. If we eat food that is *tamasic*, we become lethargic and over time may even feel depressed. On the other hand, if we eat food that is healthy and *sattvic*, we become more energetic, balanced, and healthy.

The purpose of the physical world is both: to experience life and be liberated. This is explained a little later.

19

Viśeṣāviśeṣa-liṅga-mātrāliṅgāni guṇa-parvāṇi

The different stages of progression of the qualities of nature are: non-physical, physical, indistinctive and distinctive.

Patanjali explains later that the qualities of nature come from the energy of consciousness. The four stages of creation are—non-physical, physical, indistinctive, and distinctive. The non-physical first becomes physical. Then it is indistinctive, it has no separate characteristics or features. Finally, there is differentiation and the formation of different species and physical forms.

There is a beautiful story in the *Chandogya Upanishad* that helps explain this sutra. There was a boy called Svetaketu. His father asked him to bring a fruit from the Banyan tree. When he did so, he asked Svetaketu to break it. He then asked him what he saw. Svetaketu replied that he saw some very small seeds. His father then asked him to break one of them. After Svetaketu did that, he asked him what he saw in it. Svetaketu replied that he saw nothing at all. His father then explained to him that from the very essence of that seed, which he could not see, comes this gigantic Banyan tree. He then continued, that the same invisible essence, is the Creator of this entire universe. That is our Self. We are That.

The sutra uses the words *alinga* and *linga* for non-physical and physical. In Sanskrit, the alphabet *'a'* when added to a word, gives its opposite meaning. *Alinga* means not *linga*. When the Divine or the non-physical becomes physical, the first form it takes is that of a *linga*. A *linga* is the shape of an ellipsoid, which is similar to an egg. Today, many temples have a *linga* in the shape of a rounded pillar, but the original shape of a *linga* is that of an ellipsoid or a flattened egg. This is the reason why the *linga* is held to be so sacred and used as a representation of the Divine. It is the first form the Divine took, when it became physical.

20

Draṣṭā dṛśi-mātraḥ śuddho 'pi pratyayānupaśyaḥ

The Seer is nothing but the power of seeing. Although pure, it appears to perceive through the beliefs of the mind.

The Seer or our Self, is pure consciousness. Our perception, however, is clouded by the beliefs of the mind. We do not perceive purely through the Self, but through the filter of our mind, which is why we are not able to perceive clearly.

21

Tad-artha eva dṛśyasyātmā

The Seen only exists for the liberation of the Self (Seer).

What is the purpose of this world if it is mainly suffering? Why do we need to come here and suffer? The physical world or the Seen, exists for the liberation of the Self. The importance of the world was probably explained best by Neale Donald Walsch, in *Conversations with God, Book 3*. We live in a relative world, full of dualities. There is hot and cold, high and low, light and darkness, and so on. The purpose of the relative world is to have different experiences. We cannot know what hot is, unless we experience cold. If it was hot all the time, we would not know what hot is. Basically, if we only had one experience without its opposite, that experience would soon lose all meaning. If we only experienced pleasure, then after a while pleasure would feel like nothing. We need to experience pain in order to give meaning to the experience of pleasure. It is for this reason that the concepts of heaven and hell would never work. Only experiencing pleasure or only experiencing pain, would lose meaning after some time. The relative world is important for God to experience the bliss of its own nature. In the absolute world, where there is only God and nothing else, there is no experience. In the relative world (the Seen), we experience something less than the bliss of our nature, till we are liberated and experience the full magnificence of our Divine nature. In the relative world, we have a whole range of experiences, including suffering, and then we truly appreciate and know the joy of our real nature, once we are liberated.

22

Kṛtārthaṁ prati naṣṭam apy anaṣṭaṁ tad-anya-sādhāraṇatvāt

Once that purpose is accomplished, the Seen disappears for the liberated but it continues to exist for the others, being common for them all.

The physical world disappears for the liberated because it has served its purpose for them. However, it continues to exist for others, as it is common for everyone. The physical world disappears for the liberated in the sense that it loses its illusory form. An enlightened being is able to perceive true reality. However, they may choose to continue to remain in this world after their enlightenment and help others, as many Masters have done.

23

Sva-svāmi-śaktyoḥ svarūpopalabdhi-hetuḥ saṁyogaḥ

Realization of one's own nature is caused by the union of the Creator with its own energy (creation).

The union between God and the individual (God's own energy or creation), results in realization of our true nature. Our own nature is Divine. We are not separate from God. The process of liberation or Self-Realization is to realize our eternal oneness with God. In this and the next two sutras, Patanjali is turning toward non-dualism. In the previous chapter, Patanjali described God in a dualistic manner—that God is a special soul untouched by the karmic process. We were given the impression that God is separate from us. Patanjali now shifts completely toward non-dualism. There are not two, there is only one. We are not separate from the Creator.

Patanjali is using non-dualistic language here. In non-dualism, all created matter is God's own energy. In dualism, the physical world, *Prakriti,* is a separate entity from our soul. In this sutra, Patanjali refers to created matter as God's own energy.

24

Tasya hetur avidyā

The cause of this union is ignorance.

Union is normally caused by wisdom not ignorance. However, Patanjali is going very deep here and explains this in the next sutra.

25

Tad-abhāvāt saṁyogābhāvo hānaṁ tad-dṛśeḥ kaivalyam

From the absence of ignorance, no such union takes place. This is the state of absolute oneness of the Seer.

If we are always one with God, then why don't we experience it? We don't experience it because of ignorance. Due to ignorance, we feel separate. In the absence of ignorance, no union takes place because we are then always in a state of oneness with our Creator. When ignorance arises, then the feeling of separateness arises, and we have to remove ignorance in order to experience union with God. When there is no ignorance, no union is required because we are already one with God in that state.

Patanjali uses the word, *kaivalya* in this sutra to describe the state of oneness of God. *Kaivalya* literally means absolute unity, or absolute oneness. *Kaivalya* comes from the word *kevala*, which means one, alone, only, sole, all, entire, whole. What this means is that in ultimate reality, there is only one, there is only God and God is the sole or only thing that exists. We are all part of this one Being. Our ignorance causes us to forget our oneness with God. 'Union' or reunion with God, is simply our remembering our eternal oneness with the Creator.

26

Viveka-khyātir aviplavā hānopāyaḥ

Uninterrupted discriminating perception, is the means for its removal.

How do we remove ignorance, so that we can experience our oneness with God? Through uninterrupted discriminating perception. There is a beautiful verse in the *Brihad-Aranyaka Upanishad* (1.3.28), that echoes the sentiment of this sutra:

From the unreal lead me to the real.
From darkness lead me to light.
From death lead me to immortality.

The unreal is something that does not exist, like the illusory world we live in. The real, truly exists. To go from the unreal to the real, we need discriminating perception. Patanjali explained to us in sutra 20 that our perception is limited by the beliefs of the mind. To remove our limited perception and our ignorance, we need discriminating perception. Then, we will reach the state of absolute oneness with God.

Western religions are based on a belief system. There are a set of beliefs one has to follow. There is very little room for asking questions. The yogic system is different. It is about enhancing our perception, till we reach the state of discriminating perception. In that state the veil of ignorance is removed, and we experience our unity with God.

Since ancient times, snakes were revered in this culture as a symbol of enhanced perception. Images of them were even found in the walls of some temples. This was because snakes have a high level of perception. When a person becomes enlightened, usually a snake appears. They are able the sense that person's evolved state of being. This reverence of snakes was also found in other ancient cultures.

27

Tasya saptadhā prānta-bhūmiḥ prajñā

One's wisdom in the final stages is in seven parts.

In the final stages before enlightenment, wisdom dawns on us in seven parts. At this time, *Kundalini,* our dormant energy, rises upwards from the base of our body through the spine to the crown of the head. As it rises, it passes through our seven major chakras. Each time it passes one of the seven chakras, one-seventh part of wisdom descends on us.

28

**Yogāṅgānuṣṭhānād aśuddhi-kṣaye
jñāna-dīptir ā-viveka-khyāteḥ**

By practicing the limbs of yoga, the impurities dissolve and the light of knowledge arises, culminating in discriminating perception.

Patanjali now begins to explain the limbs of yoga. By practicing the limbs of yoga, our impurities are dissolved, and the light of knowledge arises within us, culminating in discriminating perception. Patanjali uses the term 'discriminating perception' only once more, at the end of the book. When discriminating perception arises, our ignorance is removed and we are liberated.

29

Yama-niyamāsana-prāṇāyāma-pratyāhāra-dhāraṇā-dhyāna-samādhayo 'ṣṭāv aṅgāni

The eight limbs of yoga are: Yama (self-disciplines), Niyama (observances), Asana (postures), Pranayama (breath practices), Pratyahara (sensory detachment), Dharana (concentration), Dhyana (meditation), and Samadhi.

Patanjali classifies yoga into eight limbs. This is what he has been renowned for over the centuries. Each of the limbs are discussed separately.

30

Ahiṁsā-satyāsteya-brahmacaryāparigrahā yamāḥ

The Yamas (self-disciplines) are: non-violence, truthfulness, not stealing, being on the path of God, and not having unnecessary possessions.

There are five Yamas or self-disciplines. They are taken up individually. The fourth self-discipline is *Brahmacarya. Brahmacarya* is sometimes translated as celibacy. However, that is an incomplete and inaccurate description. A *Brahmacarya* is an unmarried sage or monk. *Brahmacarya* is made up of two words—*Brahman* and *carya. Brahman* stands for God and *carya* means practicing or occupied with. It essentially means, someone who is on the path of God. A *Brahmacarya* is unmarried, celibate, fully on the path of God, working on their liberation. They have chosen not to have a family, so that they can focus exclusively on their liberation. It can also pertain to married people on the spiritual path, not just those who are celibate, but normally this is a term used for unmarried, celibate monks.

31

Jāti-deśa-kāla-samayānavacchinnāḥ sārva-bhaumā mahā-vratam

These great vows apply to the entire world, and are not limited by class, place, time or circumstances.

The great vows or self-disciplines are eternal and for everyone. They should be applied by everyone, irrespective of race, religion, caste, class, or gender. They should also be practiced at all times, under any circumstances.

Three of the Yamas one can have no argument with. Truthfulness, not stealing and not acquiring unnecessary possessions, are eternal vows and stand for all time. *Brahmacarya* also needs to be taken here in a broader sense, as one who is on the path of the Divine. It cannot just be for celibate sages. If the whole world became celibate, then there would soon be no human race left. However, being on the path of God is a self-discipline that is eternal.

Some questions may arise with the first self-discipline—non-violence. Should you be non-violent in all circumstances and at all times? *The Bhagavad Gita*, one of Hinduism's most sacred texts, was taught on a battlefield. Arjuna did not want to go to war and kill his own relatives. Lord Krishna exhorts him to do his duty and fight in a righteous war. Sometimes, it is necessary for a society to go to war. Failure to do so can result in disastrous consequences. If the world had not gone to war against Hitler and allowed him to rule, the effect on the world would have been calamitous. However, one needs to make a distinction between an individual and a society. Patanjali is here, primarily concerned with the individual. An individual in their personal life should always strive to remain non-violent. However, for a society or nation, it is sometimes necessary to go to war, to protect themselves.

To be non-violent also means that one does not respond even when one is attacked. There should be no attempt to strike back, or seek revenge. One should be completely defenceless and have only good thoughts and prayers for those who try and harm us. This is very similar to the teachings of the Buddha and of Jesus Christ. Buddha taught that we should only have universal love toward those who harm us and Jesus said that we should love our enemies and bless those who curse us. He further said that if someone slaps us on the right cheek, we should offer him the left. Non-violence is a very noble idea. The principle of choosing not to harm another living being, is divine. It is practiced by highly evolved human beings and is the hallmark of any advanced civilization.

32

Śauca-saṁtoṣa-tapaḥ-svādhyāyeśvara-praṇidhānāni niyamāḥ

The Niyamas (observances) are: cleanliness, contentment, austerities, study of sacred texts, and service to God.

Niyamas (observances) are the second limb. Yamas are more social in nature. They have more to do with our conduct with others. Niyamas are more personal. They are concerned with our own individual self.

33

Vitarka-bādhane pratipakṣa-bhāvanam

On being disturbed by negative thoughts, think of their opposite.

Before proceeding further with the limbs of yoga, Patanjali is giving us practical advice on how to live our lives. When negative thoughts or emotions, such as violence, greed, anger, jealousy, etc. arise, negate them by thinking of their opposite. If you do this, those negative thoughts are immediately replaced by positive thoughts and there is no possibility of these negative thoughts being acted upon. Then, no harm can come to you or anyone else.

34

Vitarkā hiṁsādayaḥ kṛta-kāritānumoditā lobha-krodha-moha-pūrvakā mṛdu-madhyādhi-mātrā duḥkhājñānānanta-phalā iti pratipakṣa-bhāvanam

When these negative thoughts such as violence, etc. are acted on and performed, or caused to be performed, or agreed upon, they are preceded by greed, anger or delusion, which may be weak, moderate or strong. The consequences of these acts of ignorance, is endless

suffering. Therefore, think of opposite thoughts, when negative thoughts arise.

Negative thoughts are usually preceded by negative emotions, such as greed, anger or delusion. These emotions may be weak, moderate or strong. If you allow these negative thoughts to persist, then there is the possibility that these negative thoughts will be acted upon, either by yourself or through others. The consequences of those negative acts of ignorance, are immense suffering on yourself. Therefore, as soon as these negative thoughts or emotions arise, think of their opposite.

Many years ago, I experienced first-hand the truth of what this verse is saying. I had volunteered for a day, to teach yoga for a yoga institute, at a jail in Kolkata. There were a handful of us who went to teach yoga at that jail, on a Sunday morning. At the end of the program, one of the inmates came up to me and started talking. He said these yoga programs had helped him immensely. It was like giving water to a man dying of thirst. He started talking about his life and said he made one fatal mistake, and did something terrible out of anger. He seemed to hint that he had taken somebody's life. I was frozen still while he was talking. There are severe consequences to our negative actions. As soon as negative thoughts arise, it is important to break the chain of thoughts and think of opposite, positive thoughts. If we do this, we prevent actions that could bring immense suffering onto us.

35

**Ahiṁsā-pratiṣṭhāyāṁ
tat-saṁnidhau vaira-tyāgaḥ**

In the presence of one who is established in non-violence, all enmity ceases.

The word *ahimsa* is usually translated as non-violence. However, it also means not injuring, or harming anyone else. When you make a commitment to practice *ahimsa* and not harm another human being, in words or actions, your nature changes immediately. You become more gentle and you find other people also responding to you more positively. When you practice *ahimsa*, you take a giant stride in your evolution. That is why it has been given first. It is the first self-discipline, in the first limb of yoga because it is important.

A person who is established in non-violence, emits a powerful energy; an energy that brings peace amongst people that have been fighting with each other. In the presence of such a person, violence and hostilities come to an end. Nowhere was this better illustrated than by Mahatma Gandhi in Noakhali.

In October 1946, shortly before India's independence and partition, there was severe communal rioting first in Calcutta, then in Noakhali in eastern Bengal. In Noakhali (located in present day Bangladesh), the minority Hindu community was attacked, after a Muslim cleric gave a call to violence. The rioting that followed, left many Hindu men dead, women raped, and some forcibly converted and married off. Mahatma Gandhi sensed that this was a new stage of communalism in India. He decided to visit Noakhali in early November 1946, and ended up staying there for almost four months, up till the end of February 1947. Some Hindu leaders wanted a military presence in Noakhali, but Mahatma Gandhi realized that this was not a long-term solution. One had to change the hearts and minds of men. He directly took on the moral and ethical basis of communalism. He met the perpetrators of religious violence and asked them why they did it. He explained that every person has the moral right to practice their own religion as long as they do not negatively affect others. He also explained to them that such actions were against the true teachings of the Quran. He also told the majority community that it was their personal responsibility to look after their minority brethren. He showed no fear and told people to shed their fears and confront the perpetrators of violence.

Initially, some of the local Muslim priests and villagers resisted Mahatma Gandhi's visit. They dug up the roads between villages, but Mahatma Gandhi persisted. He walked barefoot from village to village in his frail seventy-seven-year-old body, spreading his message of peace and communal harmony. The effect of Mahatma Gandhi's visit was immediate and lasting. Not only did rioting end in Noakhali, but also in Bihar, where Hindus had attacked Muslims in reprisal for the riots in Noakhali. A few months later, during India's independence and partition, Bengal was spared the kind of rioting and bloodbath that occurred in Punjab, where even the presence of the military had little effect. *In the presence of one who is established in non-violence, all enmity ceases.*

36

Satya-pratiṣṭhāyāṁ kriya-phalāśrayatvam

A person established in truthfulness, receives the fruits of their actions.

A person established in truthfulness receives the rewards of their truthful actions. Patanjali explained to us in sutras 12 and 14, that our actions have consequences. Pleasure and pain are consequences, caused by being virtuous or wicked. When our actions are based on truthfulness, the consequences to us are wonderful.

Usually when we take action in this world, we face some resistance. The more we act, the more resistance or friction we face. Sometimes, people get disheartened and give up. However, when your actions are based on truth, you always succeed. Truth is like a lubricant that removes friction. You may experience some failures along the way but in the end, you will be successful. Truth always triumphs. You will receive the rewards of your work, your work will not be a failure. Whether you are starting a new venture, or working in an organisation, or doing service, your actions will always bring results when they are based on the truth. Patanjali says, you will receive the rewards of your work, your work will not go waste.

37

Asteya-pratiṣṭhāyāṁ sarva-ratnopasthānam

For one established in not stealing, all wealth approaches.

A person who does not steal, receives all wealth. Wealth here is not just material, it is also spiritual. We normally think of wealth only in material terms. However, true wealth is actually the kind of person we are and the positive impact we have on others. When you have an abundance of happiness and share that with others, that is real wealth. When you are not interested in taking from others, but only in giving of yourself, that is real wealth. We are normally in a transaction mode with other human beings. We are always trying to see what we can get. This may not be stealing, but in a way we are looking to see what we can extract from another. That is why you see so many individuals chasing rich people. They think rich people have more wealth, and therefore one can get more from them. When this sutra speaks of a person who is established in not stealing, think of not stealing in a broader sense, not only not stealing but also not wanting to only take from others. When we are not interested in taking from others, we become a person who only wants to give to others—of our time, our happiness, our service. That is real wealth.

38

Brahmacarya-pratiṣṭhāyāṁ vīrya-lābhaḥ

A person established on the path of God, gains vigour.

Spiritual practices generate a lot of energy. They make our body vibrant, healthy and strong. The benefits of practicing the next few limbs of yoga, Asanas (postures) and Pranayama (breath practices), is discussed later in this chapter. Through these practices, one gains vigour.

The word *Brahmacarya* as explained earlier, is sometimes translated as celibacy. It means someone who has controlled their sexual energies. Some translate this verse as: *A person established in celibacy, gains vigour.* The body has various types of cells. The semen is a different kind of cell. It is special. It has the power to create another life. It has a greater potency than other cells in the body. If we conserve this cell through celibacy, then the body gains vigour. If we waste it by having a lot of sex, then the body becomes weak. During major sporting events, coaches sometimes instruct their athletes, not to indulge in sex during the sporting event. Their viewpoint is the same—by abstaining from sex, the body becomes strong. When one is performing intense spiritual practices, it helps to be celibate at that time. Celibacy can make one's progress faster.

Yoga teaches us about a special non-physical form of energy, called *Ojas*. *Ojas* have many benefits. They make the body healthy and strong; they make us more peaceful and they help us progress in our journey toward liberation. The creation of *Ojas* is enhanced by spiritual practices and also by abstaining from sex.

39

Aparigraha-sthairye janma-kathaṁtā-sambodhaḥ

On perseverance of, not having unnecessary possessions, one obtains complete knowledge of the 'how and why' of birth.

When you live a simple life and do not acquire unnecessary possessions, you gain complete knowledge about birth—how and why a person is born or reborn. This knowledge involves the entire karmic process, and the reason why a soul chooses a particular family to be born in.

Aparigraha—not having unnecessary possessions or having few possessions, is the last of the Yamas, or self-disciplines. It is the self-discipline that has the most impact on the environment of our planet. The main reason our planet has suffered environmental degradation is because we consume too much. Every time we buy something, we are digging up the planet to make that product. All products require energy and natural resources, to make. When you practice this self-discipline, you will live simply and will change your car, mobile or computer, after greater intervals. You will also buy fewer products and find that you can be happy with a lot less possessions. Consequently, your life will have less impact on the environment of this planet.

Patanjali called these five self-disciplines the great vows, that stand for all time. You can see why this is so. These self-disciplines are as relevant today as they were three thousand years ago, when Patanjali wrote about them. There are billions and billions of people who have walked this planet and vanished without a trace of their work. The few who have made a lasting positive impact, have followed some or all of the self-disciplines, mentioned here. In the last century, Mahatma Gandhi and Martin Luther King Jr. were amongst a handful of people, who made a lasting impression on the world. For Mahatma Gandhi, truth and non-violence were his two most cherished values. His autobiography was titled, *The Story of My Experiments with Truth.* Others, like Martin Luther King Jr. believed and practiced some of these self-disciplines.

40

Śaucāt svāṅga-jugupsā parair asaṁsargaḥ

From cleanliness, one develops a distaste for one's own body and for comingling with other bodies.

Patanjali now starts explaining the second limb of yoga, the Niyamas (observances). Cleanliness of the body is the first practice we need to observe. From keeping the body clean, you will observe how easily it becomes dirty. If we do not wash our body for one day, it will be smelling. Then, we have the lower openings of the body that are used for excreting waste. Those parts of the body are always dirtier than the rest of the body. If you really think about it, the human body is unclean and emits a foul odour. We need to bathe it regularly, in order to keep it clean and smelling nice. When you look at the body from this perspective, you will develop a distaste for the body. This is what Patanjali is doing here, he is changing our perspective of the body. When you develop a distaste for the body, you will no longer wish to mingle or have sex with other bodies.

41

**Sattva-śuddhi-saumanasyaikāgryendriya-
jayātma-darśana-yogyatvāni ca**

And one develops purity of nature, cheerfulness, one pointedness, control over the senses and readiness for Self-Realization.

When we are no longer always thinking of sex, we develop a pure nature, we become cheerful, our mind becomes focussed, we have control over the senses and we are ready for liberation. We gain all this simply by changing our perspective of the body and developing a distaste for it, and thereby dropping our desire for sex. One of the difficulties of stilling the mind, is our attraction for sensory pleasures, particularly for sex. When we are able to overcome this, we acquire all the benefits mentioned in this sutra.

42

Saṁtoṣād anuttamaḥ sukha-lābhaḥ

From Contentment, unsurpassed happiness is obtained.

To be content means that you do not need anything outside of yourself to be happy. If you are dependent on the outside world for your happiness, then you become a slave to external conditions. If you derive your happiness from within, then you are content with your own nature. This contentment leads to unsurpassed happiness as the outside world no longer disturbs you. This does not mean that you agree with what is happening outside. You may disagree with external situations and seek to change them, but you will not need them or require them for your happiness.

43

Kāyendriya-siddhir aśuddhi-kṣayāt tapasaḥ

From practicing austerities, the impurities are removed, and the body and sense organs reach a state of perfection.

The world *tapas* means austerities. It also means heat. When you apply heat to metal, you remove the impurities, and make it pure. Similarly, austerities are yogic practices that heat the body and cleanse it from impurities. It is not that the temperature of the body rises. The body temperature remains the same but the body gets energised. You are able to perform far more activities without getting tired.

These austerities can be practiced in a number of ways. It can be done through chanting of particular mantras, performing certain breath practices (Pranayama), or dynamic practices like *Surya Namaskar* (Salutations to the Sun), and even through the food we eat. Foods like neem, turmeric and horse gram, purify and energise the body.

44

Svādhyāyād iṣṭa-devatā-samprayogaḥ

From the study of sacred scriptures, arises union with one's favourite deity.

Some sacred scriptures show us the path to union with God. That is what this text is also doing. It is showing us the way to our liberation. Studying and practicing the wisdom given in these scriptures, leads to our enlightenment.

Yoga places a lot of emphasis on learning from a Guru. Certain advanced techniques should not be learnt from books as they can cause harm, if practiced incorrectly. Having a living Master helping us, is more effective than learning from a book. Imagine if Patanjali was alive and helping us himself. Would that not be more effective than learning from a book? Of course it would. He could answer all our doubts and questions and choose a path best suited for us, based on our individual temperaments. Patanjali, for some reason, does not discuss the role of the Guru as a means for our liberation. Maybe in his time, it was difficult to travel and find a real Master.

45

Samādhi-siddhir īśvara-praṇidhānāt

From service to God, comes complete attainment of Samadhi.

Service to God (or life), brings about complete attainment of Samadhi and our liberation. No other limb of yoga is necessary.

This is sufficient for our liberation. This is such an important path, that Patanjali mentions it three times. It is mentioned in Chapter One, sutra 23 and it is also mentioned in the very first sutra of this chapter. A chapter devoted to spiritual practices, lists this first—service to God.

When you are serving God or serving life, you are putting other people's needs above yours. You understand at a deep level that your needs are always taken care of. The focus of your life is the wellbeing of others. Sometimes, an incident can change the course of your life and make you lead a life of service. It happened to Mohandas Karamchand Gandhi, later to be known as Mahatma Gandhi.

Mahatma Gandhi was educated as a lawyer in England. He was initially a very meek and mild person. In his first case in Bombay, he was so nervous when he got up to speak in court, that he found he could not say anything and had to sit down. He then informed his client to appoint another lawyer. In 1893, Gandhi relocated to South Africa, on a yearlong contract with an Indian firm, based in Natal. On June 7, 1893, he took a train from Durban to Pretoria, to attend a case for his client. He purchased a ticket in the first-class compartment. A fellow passenger complained about Gandhi's presence in that compartment, as first class was meant only for white passengers. Some railway officials then appeared and asked Gandhi to move to the Van compartment, which was meant for coloured people. Gandhi refused. He was then forcibly evicted at the next station, Pietermaritzburg. His luggage was also thrown out. He spent that cold winter night in a small, unheated waiting room at the station. His overcoat was in his luggage, but he was too scared to ask for it lest he should be insulted again.

That night at the Pietermaritzburg train platform, changed Mahatma Gandhi forever. He decided to stay back in South

Africa and fight against racial discrimination. He felt it would be cowardice to return to India, without fulfilling his obligation. He launched a movement against South Africa's discriminatory policies. Out of his movement came the concept of *Satyagraha*, which literally means, 'holding on to the truth.' *Satyagraha* employs non-violent methods to win over an opponent's mind and create a new balance between both sides of a conflict. Gandhi returned to India in 1914 and joined India's freedom movement against British colonial rule. He used *Satyagraha* against British rule and eventually helped India win its independence in 1947.

Mahatma Gandhi had a positive impact on the lives of millions and millions of people. He changed the course of world history. Apart from winning India its independence, he also had a major influence on Martin Luther King Jr. and the American Civil Rights Movement. Nelson Mandela said that Mahatma Gandhi's values of tolerance, mutual respect and unity, had a profound influence on their freedom movement and on his own thinking and they continue to inspire them, in their efforts at reconciliation and nation building. Mahatma Gandhi's life of service all began one cold winter night on a railway platform in Pietermaritzburg, on 7th June1893.

46

Sthira-sukham āsanam

Asana is a stable and comfortable posture.

Asana is the third limb of yoga. Patanjali says an Asana is a stable and comfortable posture. Traditionally, there are eighty-four important asanas in yoga. Asanas are different physical postures that one holds for a particular period of time. Asanas have many benefits. They make us flexible, they improve our health, they enable us to sit in a meditative asana (posture) for a long period of time, which is what Patanjali is most interested in. Asanas also prepare the body for higher states of consciousness. In a higher state of consciousness there is a greater flow of energy in the body. Asanas enable the body to handle a higher amount of energy.

47

Prayatna-śaithilyānanta-samāpattibhyām

By both, hardly moving and joining with the eternal.

To still the mind you have to first still the body. It is tougher to still the mind, when the body is moving. That is why a stable and comfortable posture is essential for making progress in our meditation practice. Once we are able to sit still and comfortably, we join with the eternal through our meditation.

48

Tato dvandvānabhighātaḥ

Thereafter, one is not afflicted by the dualities.

When we touch the eternal, then the dualities like pleasure and pain, no longer cause us suffering. If we touch the Divine even for a brief moment during our meditation, then there is a disconnect with the body. There is a certain gap that opens up between us and the body and we no longer identify with the body. Once that happens, the dualities cease to affect us and cause us any pain.

49

Tasmin sati śvāsa-praśvāsayor gati-vicchedaḥ prāṇāyāmaḥ

After that stable posture is maintained, regulate the flow of breath—inhalation and exhalation. This is Pranayama (breath practices).

Pranayama or breath practices, is the fourth limb of yoga. A pranayama is a certain breathing technique. You breathe in a particular way as explained in the next sutra. Some people call it breathing exercises, but they are much more than that.

Our breath and our mind are connected. When we control our breath, we are able to exert some control over our minds. If you are tense or nervous, one of the fastest ways to relax is to take a few deep, long breaths. You will find your body and mind immediately relax. Some sportsmen do this during major sporting events to relax their mind, so that they can perform at their best.

The pranayamas taught in yoga have an amazing effect on the body. The entire body is revitalized and one feels years younger. Pranayama also increases our energy levels. If we want to raise our level of consciousness, the first thing we need to do is raise our energy levels. Raising consciousness without raising energy levels is very difficult.

Each of these limbs are a vast subject on their own. There are books written on asanas and pranayama alone. People get hooked onto yoga because they feel so good once they start practicing asanas and pranayama. The entire body feels vibrant, with lots of energy, and one is more easily able to deal with life's problems. In fact, people suffering from depression are encouraged to practice asanas and pranayama, as the increase in their energy levels, brings them out of their depression.

50

Bāhyābhyantara-stambha-vṛttiḥ deśa-kāla-saṁkhyābhiḥ paridṛṣṭo dīrgha-sūkṣmaḥ

The movement of the breath is either external, internal, or stationary. It is regulated by part, time and number, and is either long or short.

Patanjali has not given us any specific pranayama, but he explains how the different pranayamas (breathing techniques) are categorised. The breath is either going out (external), coming in (internal), or it is stationary. We divide each of these breaths into parts, for a particular time and give it a number. For example, a breathing ratio that is used in some of the pranayamas is 4:16:8:4. What this means is that we breathe in for a count of 4, hold our breath for a count of 16, exhale for a count of 8 and hold again for a count of 4. Different ratios are used to revitalize different organs, or parts of the body. The pranayamas are sometimes combined with bandhas and mudras. A bandha is a lock. There are three of them—at the throat, abdomen, and the perineum. They lock energy in a particular area, and also help in spiritual awakening. Mudra is translated as 'gesture.' They are subtle physical movements that deepen our awareness. With pranayama, usually mudras which are specific hand positions, are used. It is remarkable, how by just changing the position of our hands, we can alter the flow of breath in our body.

The different pranayamas use rapid or slow breath, may use breathing ratios, combined with certain locks (bandhas), and apply hand positions or other gestures (mudras). The effect of all these pranayamas is, revitalization of the body, increase in energy levels, stillness of mind, and spiritual awakening. It is remarkable how our ancient yogis discovered all these subtle techniques, and how to combine them in different ways, so that they have a major impact on the human body, mind and energy system. Their knowledge of the working of the entire human body was at a different level.

If our body is unhealthy, then our health will take up most of our attention and we will be unable to spend time on our spiritual development. Asanas and pranayama make our body healthy, so that our body is not an impediment to our spiritual growth. Instead, it becomes a platform for our further evolution.

51

Bāhyābhyantara-viṣayākṣepī caturthaḥ

The fourth type is beyond the limits of the external and the internal.

There were three movements of breath that were discussed in the last sutra—external, internal and stationary. The fourth type is when the breath stops on its own. It's a spontaneous cessation of the breath. This can happen when one is deep in meditation. There is no practice required for this fourth type. It happens on its own, when one is ready for it. The breath may stop for a few minutes, or for a longer period of time. Normally, we would not survive if we stopped breathing. But in this advanced state, there is no negative effect on the body. The body is in a fully vibrant and stable state.

52

Tataḥ kṣīyate prakāśāvaraṇam

Thereafter, the covering over the inner light, is destroyed.

When the breath stops on its own, then the covering over our inner light, our Self, is removed. One then moves to a completely different plane of existence and a new reality unfolds.

53

Dhāraṇāsu ca yogyatā manasaḥ

And the mind becomes fit for concentration.

Then, the mind becomes ready for concentration. The mind has not fully come under our control, but its activities have substantially subsided.

54

Svaviṣayāsamprayoge cittasya svarūpānukāra ivendriyāṇaṁ pratyāhāraḥ

When the senses detach from their own objects, they seem to resemble the mind's own form. This is Pratyahara (sensory detachment).

Pratyahara (sensory detachment) is the fifth limb of yoga and a very important limb. Patanjali mentions it three times in the last chapter—sutras 12, 15, and 37. By itself it is sufficient to take one to the state of Samadhi. Why is detachment so important? The mind is constantly seeking pleasures. It is always thinking about pleasures of the senses it can enjoy, like food, sex, holidays, purchase of expensive clothes, cars, houses, and so on. This takes up a significant proportion of the activities of the mind. When you are constantly craving sensory pleasures, it becomes impossible to still the mind. It also means you are deeply identified with the body. When you are detached from the objects of the sense and no longer desire them, the mind starts becoming still.

The word *asamprayoga* used in the above sutra means, detachment, disconnected, no contact, or no joining together. A sense organ detaches, or disconnects from their own objects. For example, how do you respond when somebody abuses you? It is very easy to abuse back or even get violent. This happens when one loses awareness and control over one's emotions. Alternatively, one can practice what this sutra is teaching us. The ears can detach or disconnect from their object, which is sound. This means, one no longer hears the abuse. We ignore it or stop listening to all sounds and focus our attention inwards. When we are able to do this with all our sense organs, then the outside world ceases to have any control over us.

One of the most important Upanishads as mentioned earlier, is the *Katha Upanishad.* It is a wonderful story of a dialogue between Yama, the God of Death and Nachiketas, a young Brahmin boy. Yama explains to him that a person is attracted to two paths, the path of pleasure and the path of joy. Those who follow joy come to good and those who follow pleasure do not reach the Supreme End. He then says:

God made the opening of the senses outwards. They go toward the world outside, not to the Self within. But a wise man who desired liberation, turned and looked inwards and found his Self.

When the senses detach from their objects, our attention turns inwards. Then, the senses seem to resemble the mind's own form.

55

Tataḥ paramā vaśyatendriyāṇām

Then, there is complete control over the senses.

At this stage there is complete control over the sense organs and one is ready for the next limb of yoga.

CHAPTER THREE

VIBHŪTI PĀDA

SPIRITUAL POWERS

This Chapter can be divided in to three broad parts. First, Patanjali discusses the three remaining limbs of yoga. Then, the bulk of the chapter is on the spiritual powers one may acquire. Finally, at the end of the chapter, Patanjali discusses our liberation.

1

Deśa-bandhaś cittasya dhāraṇā

Concentration is fixing the mind to one place or object.

Concentration is the sixth limb of yoga. When we fix our attention to a particular place or object, that is concentration. The object of attention can be something external, or internal, like our breath. Initially, our attention may not be continuous. It may get broken up because our mind gets distracted by thoughts. When that happens, we need to keep bringing our attention back to the object.

Normally, our mind is dispersed. It is thinking of many different things and hopping from one subject to another.

Now through concentration, we are trying to focus the mind on one object only, without thinking.

2

Tatra pratyayaika-tānatā dhyānam

Meditation is the continuous flow of attention, on that place or object.

Meditation is the seventh limb. It is a deeper stage of concentration. When your attention on an object becomes unwavering, then that is meditation. Initially, when we are focussing on an object, there may be breaks in our flow of attention. Most people's span of attention is limited. They are unable to focus their attention on anything for long. When our attention becomes continuous, when there are no breaks, then we have reached a state of meditation.

Meditation is a natural state of progression from concentration. In concentration, there may be breaks in our flow of attention on an object. In meditation, we are able to continuously maintain our attention on the object.

3

Tad evārtha-mātra-nirbhāsaṁ
svarūpa-śūnyam iva samādhiḥ

That same meditation, when only the object appears and it seems like one's own form is non-existent, that is Samadhi.

Samadhi is the eighth and final limb of yoga. It is a natural progression from the previous limb. Patanjali defined the state of Samadhi in sutra 43 of Chapter One. He is giving the same definition here. When one is meditating there are three—the meditator, the object being meditated on, and the knowing of it. When we are in a state of meditation (the previous limb), there comes a time when the distinction between the meditator, the object being meditated on and the knowing of it, all gets mixed up and they appear one. Patanjali called this the state of Samapatti (Chapter One, sutras 41 and 42). After that, the memory gets cleansed, and it seems like one's own form is non-existent and only the object appears. That state is Samadhi. Patanjali has not discussed the state of Samapatti here, like he did in Chapter One. He goes straight from the state of Meditation (continuous flow of attention on an object), to Samadhi, where only the object appears, but obviously one passes through Samapatti to get to Samadhi.

Samadhi is the eighth and final limb of yoga. Once we reach Samadhi, have we attained liberation? Patanjali had explained in the previous chapter (sutras 26–29), that we need to remove ignorance to attain union with God. We require discriminating perception to remove ignorance and the way to acquire discriminating perception, is by practicing the eight limbs of yoga. Now that we have practiced the eight limbs of yoga and reached Samadhi, do we acquire discriminating perception and become enlightened? Not yet. In Samadhi we are very close to liberation, but there is one further decision we need to take before discriminating perception dawns on us. Patanjali explains this at the end of this chapter and at the end of the next chapter.

4

Trayam ekatra saṁyamaḥ

These three practiced together, is Samyama.

When Concentration, Meditation, and Samadhi are practiced together on an object, it is called Samyama. The last three limbs practiced together, is Samyama.

5

Taj-jayāt prajñālokaḥ

From mastery of Samyama, comes the light of wisdom.

When you give something deep attention, it opens up and reveals all its secrets. This is the basic principle behind Samyama. In the state of Samadhi, we have access to divine wisdom and intelligence as was explained to us at the end of Chapter One (sutras 48, 49). When we apply this focussed attention (Samyama), to a particular object, that object then gives us full knowledge about itself. This chapter is on spiritual powers that one can attain. We attain knowledge and these powers, by applying Samyama to different objects.

6

Tasya bhūmiṣu viniyogaḥ

Its application is to be done in stages.

Samyama is to be applied in stages to different objects.

7

Trayam antaraṅgaṁ pūrvebhyaḥ

These three—Concentration, Meditation and Samadhi, are internal limbs, compared to the preceding limbs.

The first five limbs are more external. They are connected with the outside world or with our body. The last three limbs—Concentration, Meditation, and Samadhi are internal. They are concerned with focussing our attention and stilling our mind.

The Yamas (self-disciplines)—non-violence, truthfulness, not stealing, being on the path of God and not having unnecessary possessions, are all connected with our relationship with the outside world. The Niyamas (observances)—cleanliness, contentment, austerities, study of sacred scriptures and service to God, have to do with our personal conduct and our work. Asanas work on our body and pranayama with our breath. Pratyahara is for detaching the senses from the objects of sense. These limbs are all outwards, or focussed on our body, breath and senses. On the other hand, Concentration, Meditation, and Samadhi are concerned with directing our attention continuously toward an object. They work on the mind and therefore they are considered internal, compared to the previous five limbs.

8

Tad api bahir-aṅgaṁ nirbījasya

However, these three are external limbs, of the seedless Samadhi.

However, these three are considered to be external limbs of the seedless Samadhi. It was explained at the end of Chapter One that initially Samadhi is with seed—the seed of our rebirth. This is because the impressions, or our storehouse of karma, still exists. When the impressions are destroyed, then we enter into seedless Samadhi.

9

Vyutthāna-nirodha-saṁskārayor abhibhava-prādurbhāvau nirodha-kṣaṇa-cittānvayo nirodha-pariṇāmaḥ

The appearance of the overpowering impression, which destroys all other impressions, occurs the moment after the mind is stilled. This development takes place on stilling the activities of the mind.

When we are in a state of Samadhi, after a time, another impression arises. This impression called, the 'overpowering impression', destroys all other impressions. In other words, it destroys our storehouse of karma. This overpowering impression appears the moment after the mind is stilled and once its work is completed, it destroys itself. Then, we enter seedless Samadhi, or Samadhi without any stock of karma.

10

Tasya praśānta-vāhitā saṁskārāt

Its extinguishment is activated by that impression.

The extinguishment of existing impressions is activated or caused by that overpowering impression. Extinguishment is an interesting word to use. It means to put out, like a fire, or to destroy. In legal terms, it is also means to cancel a debt. Our storehouse of karma is the fruits or consequences of our past actions, that we have to experience in the future. When we extinguish this storehouse of karma, we cancel our obligation to experience the consequences of our past actions. Then, we are totally free from our past.

11

Sarvārthataikāgratayoḥ kṣayodayau
cittasya samādhi-pariṇāmaḥ

On diminishment in thinking of many things, and rise in one-pointedness of the mind, there is development in Samadhi.

The mind normally thinks of many things and frequently moves from one subject to another. When there is a reduction in our thoughts and a rise in our ability to focus on one thing, then we progress in Samadhi.

12

Tataḥ punaḥ śāntoditau tulya-pratyayau
cittasyaikāgratā-pariṇāmaḥ

Then again, when the idea that has passed and that which has arisen is the same, that is development of one-pointedness of the mind.

Patanjali now explains the same thing in a different way. When the idea or thought that is in your mind remains the same, then the mind has become one-pointed. When the idea that passes and the idea that rises, is the same, then the mind has developed in one-pointedness.

13

Etena bhūtendriyeṣu dharma-lakṣaṇāvasthā-pariṇāmā vyākhyātāḥ

Through this, the transformations in the nature, qualities, and conditions of the elements and the senses, is also fully explained.

When we reach a state of Samadhi, there is a revitalization of the body. The nature, quality and conditions of the primary elements that make up the body, undergo a transformation. The same happens with the sense organs and the rest of the body. The entire body changes once the mind changes. When the mind becomes one-pointed in Samadhi, it has a transformative effect on the elements, the sense organs, and the rest of the body. The *Shiva Sutras* (3.38–39) says something similar:

After enlightenment, there is an infusion of vitality, beginning with the three states.

As in the states of mind, so also in the body, the sense organs, and in exterior actions.

14

Śāntoditāvyapadeśya-dharmānupātī dharmī

A living being with its individual characteristics, has a past, present and future, with its nature and qualities determined as a consequence of the preceding stage.

Each individual has their own nature, temperament and qualities. What we are today is a result of what we were in the past, whether this lifetime or previous lifetimes. Our storehouse of karma determines the kind of person we are. Our nature, our personality, how we respond to different situations, are all influenced by our storehouse of karma. Two different people will react differently to the same situation. One may get angry, and one may remain calm. This is because their nature is different. And what determines their nature? It is the karmic content stored within them. The work we do in this lifetime plays a great role in shaping the kind of human being we become. However, the work we have done in past lifetimes is stored in our storehouse of karma and it determines the type of person we are when we start off in this lifetime.

What this also means, is that our destiny is completely in our hands. We create our own future. We can do this consciously, or unconsciously. It is a result of our thoughts, words and actions. Our present nature and qualities, is a result of what we have thought, spoken or done in the past. How fast we evolve, what kind of human being we become, is completely in our own hands. It depends on how much work we put into ourselves, or how much effort we make in changing ourselves.

Our thoughts, words, and actions apart from determining what kind of person we become, also determine our life situation. As the Buddha explained in the *Dhammapada*, all that we are, is the result of what we have thought. It is based on our thoughts and is made up of our thoughts. If we speak or act with an evil thought, pain follows us as surely as the wheel of a cart follows the foot of an ox. Similarly, if we speak or act with a pure thought, happiness follows us, like a shadow that never leaves us.

15

Kramānyatvaṁ pariṇāmānyatve hetuḥ

The difference in these successive stages is the cause of the difference in evolution.

You will find different people at different stages of evolution, as a consequence of what they thought, spoke or did, in the past. The entire human race is not at the same level of evolution. We are all at different stages of evolution, based on our actions in each of the successive stages of our past.

16

Pariṇāma-traya-saṁyamād atītānāgata-jñānam

From Samyama on the three transformations (of nature, qualities and conditions), knowledge of the past and future is obtained.

For most of the next 34 sutras, Patanjali describes various Samyamas one can perform and the resulting powers and knowledge that accrue to one. Not much commentary is required for these sutras. The principle is basically the same—if you give something focussed attention, it will open up and reveal its secrets to you. In this sutra, one has to perform Samyama on the three transformations of the elements and senses.

When you read about some of the powers or knowledge,

one can obtain in the following sutras, it may appear a little far-fetched. However, there are many examples of individuals who have exhibited these powers. One such person was the Kashmir Master Vasugupta, who lived in the eighth century AD. *The Shiva Sutras* were revealed to him by Lord Shiva. He was also the author of another text, *The Spanda Karikas.* Spanda literally means vibration, throb, or movement. He said Shiva or God, is consciousness and consciousness is not inert. It has a vibration, a throb in it. It is pulsating with energy. He also said consciousness gives life to everything, and this Spanda or vibration quality of consciousness, is found everywhere in the external world. If you look at an object that is still, like a table, you may wonder where is the vibration or movement in it? On the surface there may be no movement but at the sub-atomic level there is always movement. All matter at its minutest level is composed of atoms. Atoms themselves are composed of sub-atomic particles called protons, neutrons and electrons. The protons and neutrons form a nucleus, and the electrons move around it in an orbit. The protons and neutrons themselves are composed of smaller particles called, quarks, anti-quarks and gluons. These smaller particles are constantly in motion. A table may be still on the surface, but within it, there is always some movement at the sub-atomic level. Most of what we know about sub-atomic particles, was discovered in the twentieth century, primarily in the 1970s and 1980s. However, Vasugupta was writing about it in the eighth century AD, a full 12 centuries before science validated what he was saying. He could have only discovered this by doing Samyama on an object and seeing the movement at its sub-atomic level.

Patanjali has been criticised for spending too many sutras, on these powers. However, he has a very good reason for doing this, which he explains at the end of this chapter.

17

Śabdārtha-pratyayānām itaretarādhyāsāt saṁkaras tat-pravibhāga-saṁyamāt sarva-bhūta-ruta- jñānam

A sound, its meaning and the idea of it, are sometimes superimposed on each other, causing confusion. By performing Samyama on them separately, knowledge of the speech of all living beings is obtained.

18

Saṁskāra-sākṣāt-karaṇāt pūrva-jāti-jñānam

By doing Samyama directly on the impressions, one gains knowledge of previous births.

Knowledge of our previous births is kept hidden from us. We may have had some unpleasant experiences, or some people may have been unkind to us. If the mind received information of all our previous births, it would get overwhelmed and would not be able to handle it. However, once we reach the state of Samadhi, then it is not a problem. The mind is strong enough to handle knowledge of all our prior births.

19

Pratyayasya para-citta-jñānam

From Samyama on their beliefs, one gains knowledge of another's mind.

20

Na ca tat sālambanaṁ tasyāviṣayībhūtatvāt

But that does not include the motives as that is not the object of the Samyama.

21

Kāya-rūpa-saṁyamāt tad-grāhya-śakti-stambhe cakṣuḥ-prakāśāsamprayoge 'ntardhānam

From Samyama on the form of one's body, one gains the ability to stop being perceived by others, by stopping light being reflected (from the body) to their eyes, and one becomes invisible.

How do we normally see an object? First, there has to be a source of light. This light is reflected by the object and reaches our eyes. Then, signals are sent to our brain, which analyzes the information and works out the appearance and location of that object. When we do Samyama on our body, light is absorbed and not reflected from our body and it no longer reaches the eyes of anyone near us. They are unable to see us and we become invisible.

22

Etena śabdādyantardhānam uktam

By this way, the disappearance of sound, etc, is also explained.

23

Sopakramaṁ nirupakramaṁ ca karma-tat-saṁyamād aparānta-jñānam ariṣṭebhyo vā

Karma is either manifesting or is dormant. From Samyama on these Karmas, or from portents of death, one obtains knowledge of one's death.

A yogi who is enlightened knows when he will leave his body. He has full knowledge of his death. He may not even need to do this Samyama. There are some yogis who even choose when to leave their body. When they leave their body intentionally, we say they have attained Mahasamadhi (The Great Samadhi). This is different from suicide. A person commits suicide because they are suffering. An enlightened yogi leaves their body intentionally because they have decided their work is over and it is now time to move on. A famous Master who did this was Abhinavagupta.

Abhinavgupta was one of the greatest masters of the non-dualistic tradition of Kashmir Shaivism. He is said to have authored over forty texts, of which only half are presently available. His most famous work was *Tantraloka* (Light on Tantra), a monumental text comprising 37 chapters, which is considered to be the definite text on Tantra.

He was born around the year 950 AD. He is said to have completed his final work on the winter solstice of 1015. Then, in June 1016, he and 1200 of his disciples, went into the Bhairava cave singing a devotional hymn, the *Bhairava-stotra.* They were never to be seen again. They had all consciously left their bodies and attained Mahasamadhi. The Bhairava cave still exists. It is located near a village called Beerwah, which is five miles from Magam, a town midway between Srinagar and Gulmarg.

24

Maitryādiṣu balāni

By Samyama on friendliness, etc, powers are gained.

25

Baleṣu hasti-balādīni

From Samyama on strengths, the strength of an elephant, etc., are gained.

26

Pravṛttyāloka-nyāsāt sūkṣma-vyavahita-viprakṛṣṭa-jñānam

From Samyama on the light of perception within, one acquires knowledge of the small, the concealed, and the distant.

27

Bhuvana- jñānaṁ sūrye saṁyamāt

From Samyama on the sun, knowledge of the world is gained.

28

Candre tārā-vyūha-jñānam

From performing Samyama on the moon, knowledge of the arrangement of the stars, is acquired.

29

Dhruve tad-gati-jñānam

By Samyama on the pole star, knowledge of the movement of the stars is obtained.

30

Nābhi-cakre kāya-vyūha-jñānam

From Samyama on the navel chakra, knowledge of the arrangement of the body is gained.

The navel chakra is Manipura chakra. A chakra is an energy centre. There are seven important chakras and a total of a hundred and twelve, in the body. Yoga says that energy moves in certain *nadis* or channels and there are seventy-two thousand channels in the body. At each chakra, there is a meeting of two or more channels. Manipura chakra is the only place where all seventy-two thousand channels meet. That is why when we perform Samyama on Manipura chakra, we gain knowledge of the internal arrangement of the body.

Sometimes when we chant a mantra, we are told to feel its vibration at the navel centre, or Manipura chakra. This is because if we feel it vibrating there, then its vibration will be felt throughout the body as that is the meeting place of all the seventy-two thousand channels.

31

Kaṇṭha-kūpe kṣut-pipāsā-nivṛttiḥ

From Samyama on the pit of the throat, hunger and thirst cease.

32

Kūrma-nāḍyāṁ sthairyam

From Samyama on the tortoise shaped channel, stability is obtained.

33

Mūrdha-jyotiṣi siddha-darśanam

From Samyama on the light at the top of the head, visions of realized masters are obtained.

34

Prātibhād vā sarvam

Or from Divine intuition, comes everything.

If we receive Divine intuition, then we receive knowledge of everything that we are trying to acquire through the different Samyamas. This happens either because we are liberated and are one with the Divine, or because we establish a connection with the Divine. One such example of the latter, was Srinivasa Ramanujan.

Srinivasa Ramanujan was a mathematical genius. He was one of the greatest mathematicians of the twentieth century, and possibly of all time. His work had a major impact on various branches of mathematics including, number theory, analysis, combinatorics, modular, elliptic and theta functions, amongst many others. His work also impacted other fields such as computer science and physics. He had very little formal education in mathematics and was mostly self-taught.

Ramanujan was born in 1887 in Erode, in the present-day state of Tamil Nadu, in India. In 1913, he wrote a letter to G. H. Hardy, a leading mathematician at Trinity College, Cambridge. He enclosed some of his equations. Hardy realized Ramanujan was a genius. His equations fitted into three categories: some were profoundly original; some were already known; and others were incorrect as stated. Hardy felt Ramanujan should not waste his time rediscovering what was already known and should concentrate on what was new. He invited Ramanujan to Cambridge. Ramanujan went to Cambridge in 1914 and was there till 1919.

In Cambridge, Ramanujan and Hardy collaborated and produced some great work. He made new and important discoveries. As a recognition of his work and achievements, he was elected a fellow of Trinity College and the Royal Society. However, Ramanujan kept poor health in England. There were wartime rations and Ramanujan found it difficult to get nourishing vegetarian food. Once when he was in hospital, Hardy visited him and said he had come in a taxi which had a boring number, 1729. Ramanujan replied, "No, it is a very interesting number; it is the smallest number expressible as the sum of two cubes in two different ways." ($1729 = 1^3 + 12^3$ or $9^3 + 10^3$).

Ramanujan returned to India in March 1919, in very poor health. He continued to work and produced some groundbreaking discoveries. He died a year later, on April 26, 1920, at the age of 32. Ramanujan produced about 3,900 equations in his life. He prayed often to his family Goddess, Namagiri. He said that Namagiri used to appear in his dreams and give him the formulas. He would frequently wake up at night and write down the formulas he had received. He frequently said, "An equation for me has no meaning unless it represents a thought of God." He had established a connection with his family Goddess, and he said that mathematics used to stream out from her. In the last year of his life, he did pathbreaking work in mock theta functions, which are used for work on black holes. He had done some of the mathematics for black holes, when science did not yet have any concept of black holes. His Divine intuition gave him knowledge that was far ahead of its time.

35

Hṛdaye citta-saṁvit

From Samyama on the heart, knowledge of the mind is acquired.

36

Sattva-puruṣayor atyantāsaṁkīrṇayoḥ
pratyayāviśeṣo bhogaḥ parārthatvāt
svārtha-saṁyamāt puruṣa-jñānam

The mind and the Self are completely different from each other. The belief that they are the same, is the cause of our experience. The mind exists for the Self. From Samyama on that which exists for itself (the Self), knowledge of the Self is obtained.

Patanjali is saying something important here. He repeats this message a few more times. The mind is different from the Self.

The mind here means the mind, body and ego. In short, this is our sense of being a separate person. The Self is our soul. It is pure consciousness. The mind is merely a tool for the Self. It is not the same as our Self.

37

Tataḥ prātibha-śrāvaṇa-vedanādarśāsvāda-vārtā jāyante

From this, Divine intuition, hearing, touch, vision and smell, are born.

38

Te samādhāv upasargā vyutthāne siddhayaḥ

On awakening, these powers are obstacles in Samadhi.

These powers are obstacles in our progress in Samadhi. They distract us and divert our attention back toward the world. If this is the case, then why is Patanjali spending so much time on these powers? Patanjali is being factual and methodical. At a certain stage in our evolution, these powers will arise. This is a fact. He shows us all the powers that may become available to us. We are to be indifferent to these powers. They are not the ultimate. It is only a transitory stage. We are to pass through this stage and proceed toward our liberation. If we are enamoured or attached to these powers, we will not be liberated and will fall back down. These powers prevent our consciousness from flowering. When we take an aeroplane to our destination, we first have to go to the boarding gate at the airport. The boarding gate is not our destination. It is only a transitory stage. We don't remain there. We pass through it to board the aircraft and then fly to our destination. Similarly, with these powers. They are only a transient stage. We pass through this stage on the way to our liberation.

39

Bandha-kāraṇa-śaithilyāt
pracāra-saṁvedanāc ca cittasya
para-śarīrāveśaḥ

From loosening the instrument of connection with one's body and by knowing the process of the mind, one may enter into another person's body.

For understanding the next three sutras, it is necessary to know something about the yogic physiology of the human body. According to yoga, the human body is comprised of five bodies or sheaths (*koshas*). They are:

Annamaya kosha, the food or physical body.

Manomaya kosha, the mental body.

Pranamaya kosha, the energy body.

Vijnanamaya kosha, the etheric or space body.

Anandamaya kosha, the bliss body.

The food or physical body is the outermost layer. The second body is the mental body. This is our thoughts and our mental processes. The third body is the energy body. It is made up of *prana* or life energy. It powers the physical and mental bodies, which would not be able to function without it. A computer needs hardware and software. But it also needs a power source to function. The energy body is that power source, that gives life to the physical body and the mental body. These three bodies are physical. The last two are non-physical.

The fourth limb of yoga, Pranayama (breath practices), works on the energy body. *Prana* is sometimes translated as breath, but it really means life energy. Pranayama actually means control of our life energies.

The energy body consists of five major life energies (*Pancha Pranas*). These energies are *prana, apana, samana, udana,* and *vyana.* Each of these energies have different functions. Udana and samana are discussed in the next two sutras. For this sutra, vyana is important. Vyana pervades the entire body. It controls the movement of our body, and it also coordinates the other life energies. Some yogis, when they die, leave some vyana energy in their body. The body gets naturally preserved and does not decay for weeks after their death.

Vyana life energy is the instrument of connection with our body that Patanjali is referring to in this sutra. When you gain mastery over vyana, you can loosen your connection with your body, and then by following a certain mental process (which Patanjali does not disclose), you can leave your body and enter another person's body.

There are many stories of people entering another person's body, in the past. It may have been common centuries ago, although one no longer hears of this. One of the most famous of these stories is of Adi Shankara, one of India's greatest saints, and a proponent of Advaita Vedanta (non-dualism). He is believed to have lived in the eighth century AD.

Once, Adi Shankara defeated a man called Madana Misra, in a debate. Then, his wife Sarasavani challenged him. She started asking him difficult questions on human sex and family life. She knew he would find it difficult to answer, as he was celibate, a *Brahmacharya*. Shankara asked for one month's time. Shortly afterwards, he was walking with his disciples in the forest, when they came across the body of a King who had just died. The King's name was Amarukan. Shankara then took his disciples to a cave. He told them that he was going to leave his body in the cave and enter the dead King's body. Whatever happens, they must protect his body till he returns.

Shankara entered King Amarukan's body, which then came to life, much to the joy of the Queen. He returned to the palace and learnt about human sexuality and family life. Some of the King's wise ministers realized that this was a different man in the King's body. He had suddenly become very wise and had started caring more for the people. They did not want this person to leave the King's body. So, they gave instructions to the soldiers to search the kingdom for a body that appeared to be dead. If they found one, they should cremate it immediately without asking any questions. If Shankara's original body was destroyed, he would not be able to return to his body and would be stuck in the King's body. Luckily, Shankara returned to his body, just before the soldiers reached the cave. Shankara then returned to the debate and answered all of Sarasavani's questions.

40

Udāna-jayāj jala-paṅka-kaṇṭakādiṣv asaṅga utkrāntiś ca

From mastery over the Udana life energy, the body can levitate, and one can walk over water, mud, thorns, etc, without touching them.

Udana life energy controls the area of the body above the neck, including our senses, the eyes, ears, and nose. It also coordinates our limbs, with the joints, muscles, and ligaments. Udana controls our relationship with gravity. When activated, it makes the body feel light, even though the weight of the body may remain the same. It lessens the effect gravity has on us and makes the body buoyant. When we gain mastery over Udana, gravity no longer has any effect on the body. The body can then levitate and walk over water, mud, etc., without touching them.

41

Samāna-jayāj jvalanam

From mastery over Samana life energy, one becomes radiant.

Samana life energy is located between the heart and the navel. It is responsible for the digestive system and the heart and the circulatory system. Samana also maintains the temperature of the body. When Samana is activated, one can live in extreme temperatures, without much clothing. One can see yogis in the Himalayan mountains, meditating while wearing hardly any clothes. They have activated their Samana, so outside temperatures no longer affect them. Samana is connected with the sun. When one gains mastery over Samana, one's body glows and one becomes radiant.

42

Śrotrākāśayoḥ sambandha-saṁyamād
divyaṁ śrotram

From Samyama on the relationship between the ear and space, one is able to listen to Divine sounds.

43

Kāyākāśayoḥ sambandha saṁyamāl
laghu-tūla-samāpatteś cākāśa-gamanam

From Samyama on the relationship between the body and space, and from Samapatti on the lightness of cotton, one acquires the ability to travel through space.

44

Bahir-akalpitā vṛttir mahā-videhā
tataḥ prakāśāvaraṇa-kṣayaḥ

Practice Samyama on the great liberated souls, who are in their natural state. Thereafter, the covering over the inner light is removed.

45

Sthūla-svarūpa-sūkṣmānvayārthavattva
-saṁyamād bhūta-jayaḥ

Our own gross form is constructed from the subtle elements. From Samyama on their significance, one gains mastery over the elements.

Our body is constructed from five elements—water, earth, fire, air, and space. Every object in the world is made up of these five elements, in different proportions. From performing Samyama on the significance of these five elements, one acquires mastery over these elements.

46

Tato 'ṇimādi-prādurbhāvaḥ kāya-sampat-tad-dharmānabhighātaś ca

After that, Anima and other powers appear, the body attains perfection and there is no damage to its essential quality.

After one acquires mastery over the elements, there are eight powers that appear:

Anima—the ability to make the body very small.
Laghima—the power to make the body light.
Mahima—the ability to make the body large.
Garima—the power to make the body heavy.
Prapti—the ability to reach anywhere.
Prakamya—the ability to fulfil one's desires.
Ishitva—the power to create anything.
Vashitva—control over all objects.

From mastery over the elements, the body also attains perfection. Patanjali defines bodily perfection in the next sutra. In addition, the body suffers no damage to its essential quality. This means the body does not age and remains in a state of perfection.

Patanjali explained earlier in sutra 38 that all these powers are obstacles in our journey to enlightenment. Ramakrishna also explained this to Swami Vivekananda in a beautiful way. He once called Swami Vivekananda alone to his room. He told Vivekananda that he possesses these eight occult powers, but he decided long ago that he was never going to use them, so he had no need for them. However, since Vivekananda was going to preach religion and do other things, he would like to give these powers to him. Vivekananda asked him whether these powers would help him realize God. Ramakrishna said no. Vivekananda then declined these powers. Ramakrishna was very happy with his refusal.

47

**Rūpa-lāvaṇya-bala-vajra-
saṁhananatvāni kāya-sampat**

Grace, beauty, strength, toughness and robustness, comprise perfection of the body.

48

**Grahaṇa-svarūpāsmitānvayārthavattva-
saṁyamād indriya-jayaḥ**

The grasping quality of one's nature follows from egoism. From Samyama on its significance, one gains mastery over the senses.

49

**Tato mano-javitvaṁ vikaraṇa-
bhāvaḥ pradhāna-jayaś ca**

From that, comes speed like the mind, existence, independent of the senses and mastery over primary matter.

50

Sattva-puruṣānyatā-khyāti-mātrasya sarva-bhāvādhiṣṭhātṛtvaṁ sarva-jñātṛtvaṁ ca

Only for one who perceives the difference between the mind and the Self, does the state of omnipotence and omniscience arise.

Patanjali repeats what he said in sutra 36—the mind and the soul are different. Only when one perceives this difference, does the state of being omnipotent and all-knowing arise. Omnipotence here is used in the sense of being the governing, or chief ruler of all beings. Omniscience in this sutra refers to knowledge of the illusory world. It does not refer to true knowledge, arising from discrimination.

51

Tad-vairāgyād api doṣa-bīja-kṣaye kaivalyam

From detachment to even that, the seed of deficiency is destroyed, and one attains liberation.

When there is no interest in even being the ruler of the world, then one is liberated. When an individual has a detachment to all the world has to offer, one attains enlightenment.

The *Katha Upanishad* also says something similar. Nachiketas had been sent by his father in anger to Yama, the God of Death. He waited for three nights without food, for Yama. For having kept him waiting without hospitality, Yama offered him three boons. The first two boons asked by Nachiketas was easily given by Yama. The third boon asked by Nachiketas was, "What happens to a man after he dies? Does he exist, or does he not exist?" Yama is hesitant to answer him. He instead offers him land and gold, and to make him a ruler of the world. But Nachiketas is insistent. He says that all these pleasures pass away, and a man cannot be satisfied with wealth. How can we enjoy wealth with him, Yama the God of Death, in sight? Yama is pleased with his reply, and then proceeds to answer Nachiketas' question.

52

Sthānyupanimantraṇe saṅga-smayākaraṇaṁ punar-aniṣṭa-prasaṅgāt

On receiving an invitation from celestial beings for intercourse, one should not accept, nor be proud as there is the possibility of falling back into the undesirable.

Shortly before enlightenment, one may be approached by celestial beings for sex. One should not accept nor be proud that they have been approached. If one accepts, it means one is still attached to bodily pleasures. If one becomes proud, then it strengthens the ego. In either case, there is the danger of falling and losing some of the progress one has made on the road to liberation.

Something similar happened to the Buddha just before his enlightenment. The demon, *Mara the Tempter*, sent his three beautiful daughters to Siddhartha Gautama, the night before his enlightenment. They stripped in front of him and tried to entice him. However, Gautama remained unmoved. The next morning, Gautama attained enlightenment and became the Buddha.

53

Kṣaṇa-tat-kramayoḥ
saṁyamād-viveka-jaṁ jñānam

From Samyama on a moment and its successive moments, comes knowledge arising from discrimination.

Time is also part of the illusion. There is only the eternal moment of Now. When you perform Samyama on time, you are able to see through the illusion. You gain knowledge born from discrimination. You are able to discriminate between what is real and unreal.

54

Jāti-lakṣaṇa-deśair anyatānavacchedāt
tulyayos tataḥ pratipattiḥ

From seeing no separable difference by race, attributes or part, compared to two objects of the same kind, arises knowledge.

Patanjali is now focussing again on non-dualism. If you look at two objects that are completely different from each other in terms of race, attributes or part, like a dog and a cat, and you find no difference between them, compared to two objects that are of the same kind, such as two dogs of the same breed, then true knowledge has arisen. How can this be possible, one may ask? We are actually living in an illusory world, where objects appear different and separate from each other. There is actually no difference, we are all one, we are not separate from each other, and we are all made from the same energy.

The *Ashtavakra Gita* puts it beautifully:

Realizing the Self is in all beings and all beings are in the Self, brings about the birth of the enlightened sage. It is strange that the intelligent man continues to exist in 'mine-ness'(3.5).

"I am in all beings and all beings are in me." This is true knowledge. Therefore, there is nothing to give up, nothing to hold and nothing to dissolve (6.4).

You are in whatever you see. Just you alone. Do bracelets, armlets and anklets of gold, appear different from gold? (15.14).

You may wonder, how can two different objects be the same? This is because all objects are made from the same thing—they are all composed from the same energy of God. There is only one soul or Self that permeates everything, as the *Ashtavakra Gita* explains. Bracelets, armlets and other jewellery made of gold, may look different from each other but they are all still composed of gold. Similarly, we all appear separate and different from each other, but we are still composed of the same thing.

The word *pratipatti* has been translated here as knowledge. It also means perception. Both meanings can be applied here. You are able to perceive the truth of two separate objects, when you realize there is no separable difference between them.

55

Tārakaṁ sarva-viṣayaṁ sarvathā-viṣayam
akramaṁ ceti viveka-jaṁ jñānam

This knowledge arising from discrimination, is liberating. It covers all regions and all objects and happens in an instant.

This true knowledge arises from discrimination. We are able to discriminate the real from the unreal. Like *Alice's Adventures in Wonderland*, we are presently living in a make-believe world, where things are not what they seem.

This discriminating knowledge is liberating. It breaks through the illusion and allows us to see clearly. We move to another dimension of existence. This knowledge covers all regions and objects and happens in an instant.

56

Sattva-puruṣayoḥ śuddhi-sāmye kaivalyam iti

When the purity of the mind becomes equal to that of the Self, there is liberation.

The mind becomes as pure as the Self when the ego has gone. When there is no trace of the ego, then the mind is as pure as the Self and one is liberated. When our individuality is obliterated, we become enlightened.

Union with God is not a meeting of two, it is a meeting of one. We do not meet God, embrace God and then become one with God. When the ego disappears, the state of God appears in us.

There is a beautiful verse in the *Brihad-Aranyaka Upanishad* (31–32) that explains the state of *Kaivalya* or liberation:

Where there seems to be another, there one may see another, one may smell another, one may taste another, one may speak to another, one may hear another, one may think about another, one may touch another and one may know another.

But when one becomes clear like water, the Seer is alone and there is no other.

The state of being alone (*Kaivalya*), is the title of the next chapter.

CHAPTER FOUR

KAIVALYA PĀDA

LIBERATION

The fourth chapter is titled *Kaivalya. As* explained earlier, Patanjali uses the word *Kaivalya*, for liberation, which is a non-dualistic way to describe liberation. The literal meaning of *Kaivalya* is absolute unity or absolute oneness. *Kaivalya* is derived from the word *Kevala*, which means alone, only, sole, one, entire, whole, all. In the liberated state, there is only One, there is only God and nothing else exists. Everything is a part of God. What this means is, that after liberation we experience our oneness with God, or with Everything. That also means that we identify with nothing, or no-thing in particular; not our mind, body or any limited thing. This is the reason why when the Buddha was asked about liberation, he said after liberation we become nothing. Some of his disciples found this hard to understand but he was describing the state of *Kaivalya*. When you become everything, then you also become nothing. *Kaivalya* is the state of liberation where we merge into the Oneness.

1

Janmauṣadhi-mantra-tapaḥ-samādhi-jāḥ siddhayaḥ

The spiritual powers arise from birth, herbs, mantras, austerities or Samadhi.

The previous chapter described various powers that arose from the practice of Samyama, which is the process of Concentration, Meditation and Samadhi, the last three limbs of yoga. The powers arise when we are in a state of Samadhi. In Samadhi our mind is still and focussed and that is when an object yields and reveals its secrets.

This sutra says, there are other ways by which we can acquire these powers. We may have these powers from birth. This means we were a highly evolved person in our previous life and had acquired the powers then. In this lifetime we do not lose our level of evolution. We start from where we ended in our previous life, which is why these powers are with us from birth.

We can also acquire spiritual powers from herbs, mantras, and austerities. One does not hear about acquiring powers from herbs anymore, and maybe that process has been lost. Austerities here refers to penance. One performs a certain penance to gain these powers. Chanting of mantras is also a powerful process. However, mantras are mainly used to attain liberation.

It should be understood that the herbs mentioned in this sutra are not in any way connected to the recreational drugs that became fashionable in the 1960s and 70s and that are still prevalent in our society today. These drugs have no value to a spiritual aspirant. This was a lesson that was made clear to Ram Dass. Ram Dass was originally Dr. Richard Alpert, a professor of Psychology at Harvard University, in the 1960s. He was very successful and had everything most people desire—lots of money, a Mercedes Benz car, a sailing boat, and a Cessna airplane. But somehow he was not fulfilled. He felt the field of Psychology did not adequately grasp the human condition. He, along with a few other Harvard professors, experimented with psychedelic drugs, particularly LSD. He found LSD gave him a high and made him feel good but he was not able to maintain that state. Invariably, there was a fall and one left that state and felt even more depressed when one came back to normal. Dr. Alpert lost his job at Harvard for consuming these drugs. However, he did not stop experimenting with them. He felt there could be a missing link that would show us how to remain in that state. He thought maybe a holy man could explain what was missing.

Ram Dass travelled to India in search of a holy man who 'knows' and could explain what was missing. By chance in India, he met another American who took him to his Guru, Neem Karoli Baba. Neem Karoli Baba was an enlightened master. The first time they met he told Ram Dass/Dr. Alpert that he had thought of his mother last night, who had died a year ago of a spleen disorder. Ram Dass was shocked. He had thought of his mother last night, who had died a year ago of a spleen disorder but he had told nobody about it. When they met the next morning, Neem Karoli Baba shouted at him when he was approaching, "Have you got a question?" Before he could reply he asked him to show him his 'medicine'. Ram Dass gave him one pill of LSD. He kept his hand extended and took a second and a third pill. He swallowed all three pills together, which was a very high dose of LSD. Ram Dass waited expectantly to see the reaction. However, nothing happened! Neem Karoli Baba remained just the same. LSD had no effect on him even though he had taken such a potent dose. Neem Karoli Baba through his actions gave a message to Ram Dass—these drugs are worthless and a waste of time. They are of no value to a spiritual aspirant and do nothing to improve the human condition. What Ram Dass was looking for, could only be found within himself.

Ram Dass spent a few months at Neem Karoli Baba's ashram. There, he was taught yoga and was also imparted the teachings of this text—*The Yoga Sutras*. Once, when he was with Neem Karoli Baba, the master touched him on his forehead three times. He immediately went into an exalted state. Tears started streaming down his face and he had to be carried out of the room.

Ram Dass returned to America. He described his experiences in his bestselling book, *Be Here Now*. Through Ram Dass, Neem Karoli Baba opened a doorway to the world. A doorway through which millions of people could learn more about yoga and could experience the benefits of a state of higher consciousness.

2

Jāty-antara-pariṇāmaḥ prakṛty-āpūrāt

The change into a different kind at birth, is for satisfying the desires of one's nature.

Patanjali had discussed karma briefly in Chapter Two, sutras 12–14. In the next few sutras, he explains how karma works.

This is a difficult sutra to translate. Most translators struggle with it. However, it is a very important sutra. It explains a key element in how karma works. The two key words to understand in this sutra are, *jāti* and *āpūra*. *āpūra* literally means flooding, filling up, making full. It is derived from the verbal root *āpṛī*, which means all of the above, and also means to satiate or satisfy one's desire. This is the meaning that Patanjali is using here—for satiating or satisfying one's desires.

Jāti as explained in sutra 2.13 means kind, class, race, species, caste. Some people translate *jāti* to means species, and believe we change into different species at birth, depending on our actions in this lifetime. However, this is not what Patanjali is saying. For him *jāti* means class, kind, or type. For example, say we have a desire to be a great leader of men. Or we have a desire to be a great tennis player. Then, in our next lifetime, we will become that type or kind of person, with the necessary qualities, to become a great leader or a great tennis player. So, what this sutra is saying, is that we change into a different type of person at birth, so that we can satisfy our unfulfilled desires.

Patanjali has also said earlier in sutra 2.13, that we are born as a particular kind of person, as a consequence of our past actions. Therefore, the type or kind of person we are at birth, is a result of two factors—our unfulfilled desires and the consequences of our past actions.

3

Nimittam aprayojakaṁ prakṛtīnāṁ
varaṇa-bhedas tu tataḥ kṣetrikavat

The motive is not the cause of nature choosing a particular kind, but then, it acts like a cultivator.

The motive behind the desire does not cause nature to choose a particular kind of human being. Continuing with the example given in the last sutra, say the motive behind becoming a great leader, was to be famous. The motive of being famous does not determine the kind of person you become in your next lifetime. It is the desire itself, to be a great leader or tennis player, that determines the kind of person you are in your next birth.

At the same time, the motive acts like a cultivator or farmer. A cultivator grows crops. In the same way, a motive grows desires. Due to this motive, we keep having more and more desires. If our motive is to be famous, then it breeds various desires to fulfill that motive. Being a great leader or tennis player is one of them. There will be more desires as long as the motive is still there.

4

Nirmāṇa-cittāny asmitā-mātrāt

Minds are created entirely from ego.

The mind and the ego are the same thing. The mind is created entirely from the ego. An alternative way to translate this sutra is, "Created minds are nothing but ego." What Patanjali is trying to say, is that the mind and the ego are virtually the same thing. That is why when you still the mind, the ego disappears, and the state of God appears. In the second and third sutras of Chapter One, Patanjali explained to us that when we still the activities of the mind, the Seer abides in its own nature. We normally identify with the body and mind. We believe we are a separate individual, which is our ego. Patanjali called this *asmitā*, 'I-ness.' As soon as we still the mind, the ego vanishes, and we no longer identify with the body and mind.

5

Pravṛtti-bhede prayojakaṁ cittam ekam anekeṣām

There is one mind of the many, that is responsible for the manifestation of variety.

One mind among the many is real. It is the mind of God. The rest are all artificial minds created by the ego. The mind of God, which is Divine intelligence, is responsible for the creation of this universe, and the variety that we see in it.

6

Tatra dhyāna-jam anāśayam

Among them, those born from meditation have no stock of karma.

Karma is of three kinds—*Sanchita, Prarabdha,* and *Agami*. *Sanchita* is our entire storehouse of karma. *Prarabdha* is the amount of karma taken from that storehouse and allotted to us to exhaust in this lifetime. *Agami* is the new karma we build up through our actions in this lifetime.

Minds that are born of meditation have no stock of karma. Patanjali is now explaining in the next few sutras, how karma is built up. He mentioned it briefly in Chapter Two. The beginning of Chapter Two described five afflictions that cause suffering. The first two are most important—ignorance and egoism. Patanjali then explained in sutra 2.12, that our storehouse of karma has its root in these afflictions. Karma depends on what our actions are based on. Are we acting from a state of awareness, or from our ego? When we act from a state of awareness, our actions do not have consequences and do not build a stock of karma. In fact, when we act from awareness, our karma is dissolved rapidly. When we act from our ego, actions have consequences and create karma. A mind that is born from meditation will act from a state of awareness. This mind will have no stock of karma.

You can see whether you act consciously or react out of habit. If somebody abuses you, it is easy to react compulsively and abuse back. It takes a great deal of consciousness, not to abuse back and to remain peaceful. When you act from a state of awareness, your actions change completely. They are no longer reactions but conscious actions.

7

Karmāśuklākṛṣṇaṁ yoginas tri-vidham itareṣām

The actions of a yogi are neither white nor black. For the others, it is of three kinds.

The actions of a yogi are neither white nor black. They are neither pure nor impure, nor are they good or bad. For others, their actions are of three types—white, black, or something in between. This means they could be good, bad, or between the two.

A yogi does what is required. His actions are neither good nor bad as he has transcended both. His actions flow from a state of awareness. They are based on what the situation requires. He or she will never refrain from doing what is required. Most of us use our actions to get to a state of being, or we act only for our personal benefit. We go on holiday, so that we can be peaceful. We do things we like, so that we can be happy. We do not enjoy going to a hospital to treat a family member. This was best explained in *Conversations with God Book 3*. *Conversations with God* says that most people have the Be-Do-Have paradigm in reverse. The believe if they 'have' a thing (more time, money and so on), they can 'do' a thing (go on a vacation, take up a hobby, buy a new home), which will enable them to 'be' a thing (happy, peaceful, or content). The creative power of the universe actually works the other way. 'Havingness' does not produce 'beingness'. It is the other way around. We first move to a state of "being"—happy, peaceful, content, love, aware. We then "do" things from that state of being and we find out that what we are doing ends up bringing us things we always wanted to "have". This is the correct way to use the creative force of the universe.

When our state of being depends on what we are doing, or is based on something external, then it is always temporary. When what we are doing changes, then our state of being also changes. However, when we reach a state of being through our effort, or our decision to be in a certain way, then it remains permanent, and what we are doing becomes a reflection of the state of being we have reached.

Beingness is its own reward. The quality of our life depends on what we are being, not on what we are doing or having. When we reach certain exalted states of being, our life becomes rich and rewarding and we no longer look to what we are doing or having, to bring meaning into our lives. Using 'doingness' to reach 'beingness' invariable builds karma. However, the reverse does not add karma. Actions flowing from a high state of being we have reached, does not build karma.

A yogi has already reached a conscious state of being. They are aware, peaceful, and happy. They act from that state of being. Their actions do not add any karma. Because they are aware, they are no longer identified with the body. They do not see themselves as the 'doer.' It makes no difference to them whether they need to go to the hospital, or on a vacation. They act from a state of consciousness and are in sync with life. They are also not looking for any personal reward or ego gratification. Their minds are not calculating, "What do I gain or lose out of this?" Their actions serve the greater good.

A householder has duties and responsibilities to their family members. They need to look after their children, parents, and spouse. So which category do their actions fit into? Actions based on one's duty to one's family or in one's workplace, or to society, do not build karma. Actions based on selfish desires, create karma. Arjuna was told in the battlefield by Lord Krishna, that it was his duty to fight in a righteous war. Actions based on one's duty are liberating and do not bind one.

8

Tatas tad-vipākānuguṇānām
evābhivyaktir vāsanānām

Thereafter, the consequences of past actions, stored as impressions, will manifest only at a suitable time.

When we are taking actions unconsciously, or from an ego, then the consequences of our actions are stored as impressions. These consequences will manifest at a suitable time, in this lifetime or the next. As explained in Sutra 2.14, the consequences will be pleasurable or painful, depending on whether one has been virtuous or wicked.

9

Jāti deśa-kāla-vyavahitānām apy ānantaryaṁ smṛti-saṁskārayor eka-rūpatvāt

Though separated by birth, place and time, there is continuity because memory and impressions are the same in form.

The impressions can manifest at a future lifetime, even though there is a separation by birth, place and time. This is because impressions are a form of memory. They continue from one lifetime to the next.

10

Tāsām anāditvaṁ cāśiso nityatvāt

The impressions have no beginning because desires have been in existence for eternity.

The question may arise, "When did the process of karma begin?" Patanjali answers that in this sutra. The impressions have no beginning because they are linked to desires, and desires have been in existence for eternity. Most of our desires come from the ego. When our actions are based on desires of the ego, then those actions have karmic consequences. In other words, those actions build up a stock of karma, called impressions.

When you think about it, it seems a little strange. We come into this world with nothing and we leave with nothing. The only thing we take with us is our karma. We build up karma because we desire things of this world. And those 'things', we cannot take with up when we pass away. Also, all objects of this world are just made up of the five primary elements in different proportions. A diamond which is valuable and mud which is worthless, are both composed of the five elements—water, earth, fire, air and space, in different amounts. We toil year after year for all these material objects, which we leave behind when we pass away, and all that effort only builds up karma, which is the only thing we take with us. The *Shiva Sutras* says something similar (3.40):

Due to desire moving outwards for external objects, an individual is carried from life to life.

11

Hetu-phalāśrayālambanaiḥ saṁgṛhītatvād eṣām abhāve tad-abhāvaḥ

The impressions are held together and sustained through the interconnectedness between the motive for an action and its consequence. On their disappearance, the impressions also disappear.

Patanjali finally gets to the heart of the matter and explains how karma is formed and what holds it together. There is a connection between the motive for an action and its consequence. If an action is based on a selfish motive, then that action has consequences (karma), which are stored as impressions. When there is no selfish motive for our actions, then our actions do not have consequences; that is, they do not build up karma, and our storehouse of karma also gets dissolved. The motive or reason behind an action, is the key. This is what determines whether an action builds up karma or not. If our motives are based on our ego and our likes and dislikes, then our actions will build karma. When our motives are pure, or when we act from a state of awareness, then our actions do not cause karma and our stock of karma (the impressions) also disappears.

Patanjali has explained in very simple terms, how to be free from the karmic process. Change the motive behind our actions. When our selfish motives disappear, then our karma also disappears. Now, you will understand why Patanjali emphasized service to God, in Chapter Two. When you lead a life of service, your actions are for the greater good, not just for yourself. The motive for your actions is for serving God and for improving the lives of others. Such actions dissolve karma, they do not accumulate karma.

At the beginning of Chapter Two, Patanjali explained the five afflictions: ignorance, ego, attraction (liking), aversion (disliking), and tenacity of mundane existence. He also said in verse 2.12 that the storehouse of karma has its roots in these afflictions. When we have an ego, we have likes (attraction) and dislikes (aversion). When our actions are based on our likes and dislikes, then our actions build karma. To set karma aside, take action according to what is required or needed in any given situation, not on our likes and dislikes.

How else do we put what Patanjali is saying into practice? What should our motives be toward our work for example, so that we are free from karma? Lord Krishna explains this in Chapter Two of the *Bhagavad Gita* (2.47, 48). These verses were also quoted in the commentary to the first sutra of Chapter Two. He said you have a right only to your work, not at any time on its reward. Do not let the rewards be the motive for your actions. Focus on the work, not on its reward. The reward will take care of itself. He also said, give up selfish desires while performing actions and be the same in success and failure. This is how one is established in yoga.

What this also means is that we live in the present moment and give full attention to the action itself. We are not attached to the results. We are fully involved in our work, making improvements and coming out with innovations, without worrying about the future. Our attention should be on the next step, not the goal. If we focus only on the goal and not the immediate step we need to take, then we will never reach our goal. In this way, we act from a state of consciousness, not from the worrying mind. The state of awareness is of primary importance. What we do is secondary. When we attain this state of awareness, we experience a certain stillness, a peace, which becomes joy. This is the peace of yoga Lord Krishna is referring to. In this state, we have already succeeded, and we no longer look to the outside world for gratification. Success or failure no longer troubles us.

The simplest way to be free of the karmic process is to serve life, to stop liking and disliking, or to act from a conscious state of being. When we are aware, we do not build any new karma and dissolve our existing karma rapidly.

12

Atītānāgataṁ svarūpato
'sty adhva-bhedād dharmāṇām

The past and the future exist in their own form. This is due to a break into parts, in the journey of the established order of things.

This chapter is titled *Kaivalya*, which means liberation and also means absolute oneness. In the next six sutras, Patanjali is speaking about the dimension of oneness. Some of what he says is difficult to understand because he is speaking from a different dimension of existence. This is a dimension we will experience once we are liberated. It is difficult to express it in words.

The past and the future already exist in a different form. We have in fact multiple futures. Which future will manifest, depends on the actions we take now. The journey of our Self is broken up into these parts.

13

Te vyakta-sūkṣmā guṇātmānaḥ

Whether manifested or unmanifested, they have the qualities of the Self.

Our present has already manifested and our future has yet to manifest. It is either in the physical state or the non-physical state. Whatever state they are in, they have the qualities of our Self. Our Self or our soul, is God. Everything exists within God. This is why all states have the qualities of the Self.

14

Pariṇāmaikatvād vastu-tattvam

The reality of objects is due to their transformation from oneness.

An object is part of God. It is transformed from that oneness and appears as a separate object. This process was explained in sutra 2.19:

The different stages of progression of the qualities of nature are: non-physical, physical, indistinctive, and distinctive.

15

Vastu-sāmye citta-bhedāt tayor vibhaktaḥ panthāḥ

Due to the mind dividing the sameness of objects, the path of these two appears different.

All objects are composed of the same energy of God and the three qualities of nature. They may appear different and look separate, but they are all part of God. The mind is like a cutting instrument. Our intellect divides all objects into separate parts. The mind sees division but our soul sees One. The mind divides the oneness of objects, which is why the path of two objects appears different.

16

Na caika-citta-tantraṁ vastu tad-apramāṇakaṁ tadā kiṁ syāt

And nor does an object's existence depend on a single mind. Otherwise, what would be the proof of that object, in its absence?

An object's existence does not depend on a single mind, otherwise in the absence of that mind, there would be no proof of its existence.

17

Tad-uparāgāpekṣitvāc cittasya vastu jñātājñātam

An object is known or unknown, depending on the mind's colouring of it.

How do you differentiate and know an object when it is part of one Whole? In ultimate reality, everything is one. Imagine a large painting running along an endless corridor. The painting has millions of objects in it. The only problem is that the painting is white and black. It is mostly white, with a few outlines in black. It is very difficult to see an object in it. Now, if you colour an object in that painting, you will be able to see it clearly. That is what the mind does. In the huge canvas of life, with an infinity of objects in it, we see an object when the mind colours it and makes it known. The object then appears as a separate entity and not as an invisible part of God. An object becomes known because our mind focuses on it. If our mind does not direct its attention on it, then it remains unknown.

18

Sadā jñātāś citta-vṛttayas tat-prabhoḥ puruṣasyāpariṇāmitvāt

The activities of the mind are always known to its master, the soul, due to the soul's unchanging nature.

In the next few sutras, Patanjali looks at the difference between the mind and our soul (Self). The soul is the master of the mind and is always aware of its activities. The soul is still, it is not changing like the mind. It is therefore able to perceive the mind clearly. When we are moving, it is difficult to see something properly. When we are still and unchanging, then we can see clearly.

19

Na tat svābhāsaṁ dṛśyatvāt

Nor is the mind self-illuminating because it is an instrument of the soul.

The mind is not self-illuminating like the sun. It is more like the moon that reflects the sun's light. The mind is an instrument of the soul. Whatever limited intelligence it has, comes from the soul. Just as the moon does not have its own light source and is only seen because of the light of the sun, in the same way the mind does not have its own intelligence, but gets its intelligence from the soul. The soul on the other hand, is self-illuminating. It has its own intelligence and is its own master.

20

Eka-samaye cobhayānavadhāraṇam

And it cannot know both simultaneously.

The mind is unable to know both, the subject and the object simultaneously. It can only know one at a time. To know both simultaneously, one needs awareness. The soul has awareness, so it is able to perceive the subject and object at the same time. The mind is basically thought, intellect and memory. It does not have the capacity to perceive both, subject and object together. This is another important difference between the mind and the soul.

21

Cittāntara-dṛśye buddhi-buddher atiprasaṅgaḥ smṛti-saṁkaraś ca

One mind being an object of another mind, would imply one intellect governing another, which is unworkable. And there would also be a mixing up of memory.

One mind cannot be the instrument or object, of another mind. That would mean one intellect governing another, which is not workable. Also, the memories of both the minds would get mixed up and we would not know which mind is which. Therefore, a mind can only be an instrument of the soul. It cannot be an instrument of another mind.

22

Citer apratisaṁkramāyās tad-ākārāpattau svabuddhi-saṁvedanam

When there is no intermixing of thoughts; when that state of mind appears, one's own intelligence becomes known.

There is no intermixing of thoughts when the mind becomes still and one-pointed. At that time, when the noise of the mind has stopped, the intelligence of our soul becomes known. Patanjali described this intelligence in sutra 1.49. He said there that this wisdom because of its extraordinary sense, belongs to a different realm from the wisdom heard from scriptures.

23

Draṣṭṛ-dṛśyoparaktaṁ cittaṁ sarvārtham

The mind that is coloured by the Seer and the Seen, knows everything.

The mind is coloured by the Seer and the Seen, when it becomes still. It then gains access to the wisdom of the Seer or our soul as explained in the last sutra. This mind knows everything because the Seer knows everything and this mind has gained access to the Seer's knowledge. It is really the Seer that knows everything. A still mind can tap into the knowledge of the Seer. Today, there is vast amounts of information on the internet. We are able to access this information with a good internet connection and device. A still mind is something like that. It accesses the knowledge of the Seer.

24

Tad-asaṁkhyeya-vāsanābhiś citram
api parārthaṁ saṁhatya-kāritvāt

However, the mind with its varied and innumerable latent impressions, exists for the sake of another (the soul) because it can only act by being in contact with it.

However, Patanjali reminds us that the mind is only an instrument of the soul and exists for the sake of the soul. It has no power of its own and can only act by being in contact with the soul. The mind also carries with it innumerable latent impressions, which is our stock of karma.

25

Viśeṣa-darśina ātma-bhāva-bhāvanā-vinivṛttiḥ

For one who sees the difference between the mind and the Self, the idea of the mind being the Self, disappears.

In the past few sutras, Patanjali has been explaining the difference between the mind and our Self (soul). The mind has to be taken in a broader sense. The mind is created entirely from ego, or is nothing but ego, as sutra 4 explained. This mind is therefore also our ego, or our identity as a separate person. We identify with this separate person and believe this is who we really are. Patanjali has explained that is not our real self. Our real Self is our soul and not the individual person, who we think we are. The *Shiva Sutras* says the same thing—*The individual self is the mind* (3.1).

You may wonder why is all this important? What has this got to do with the eight limbs of yoga, or the state of samadhi that Patanjali has spent time on in the previous chapters? Well, Patanjali is giving us a new and easy way to be enlightened. He is changing our perception. We are in a state of ignorance because we are identifying with our mind and our body, or our individual identity. He has painstakingly explained to us that the mind is only an instrument of the Self, which is the true life within us. When we understand the difference between the mind and the Self, then we no longer identify with the mind and body, but with the Self.

It should be understood that a person who has attained Samadhi knows fully well the difference between the mind and the Self. Their mind is still and they are completely identified with the Self.

26

Tadā viveka-nimnaṁ kaivalya-prāgbhāraṁ cittam

Then, the mind becomes inclined toward discrimination and is close to liberation.

Then the mind becomes inclined toward discrimination between the real and the unreal and one is close to liberation. Normally, we are lost in the activities of the mind. How much attention do we give to the basic life force, our Self, that breathes life into our body and mind? Without the Self, neither the body nor the mind could exist. When we no longer identify with the mind, then our mind automatically turns inwards and focuses its attention on the Self.

When we are identified with our mind and body, we accumulate a whole lot of other identities, which may be based on our education, wealth, race, religion, nationality, status in society, and so on. We identify with our wealth, or our education, or our nationality. All these identities are false. At the time of our death, these are stripped away automatically. When we understand and practice what Patanjali is teaching us here, we drop all these identities. We become a life without any false accumulations. We are encouraged to do this at Mount Kailash. When we go on a pilgrimage to Mount Kailash, the circumambulation of the mountain starts just after Darchen, at the shrine of *Yamadwar*. Yamadwar literally means, 'the doors of the God of Death.' At Yamadwar, we are to drop our identification with our physical body and just be consciousness, or a life with no false identities. We drop our physical self and align with our spiritual self as we are going to meet Lord Shiva.

In sutra 1.36, Patanjali had also asked us to direct our attention on our Self. A great way to do this is simply to focus our attention on our breath. Our breath is the basic life force of the body. Without the breath our body cannot survive. In the *Vigyan Bhairava Tantra*, Lord Shiva gives 112 meditations for our liberation. At the end of the text he gives one more meditation, which he says is easy for anyone to practice. That meditation is listening to the sound of one's breath.

27

Tac-chidreṣu pratyayāntarāṇi saṁskārebhyaḥ

During breaks in that state, other ideas may arise due to latent impressions.

There will be breaks in that state where we are focussing our attention on the Self. During those breaks other ideas will arise due to our latent impressions. These impressions are our storehouse of karma, which has made us into a particular kind of person. Karma is our memory. It shapes who we are as a person. We have certain habits because of karma. The spiritual process works to remove the influences of these impressions or memories from our lives. Due to these memories, ideas arise and we once again identify with our mind and body, or with certain aspects of our life. Old habits arise again. We may identify with the education we have had, the recognition we achieved in our work, the country or race we belong to, the profession we practice, or many other things.

28

Hānam eṣāṁ kleśavad uktam

These can be removed just like the afflictions, explained earlier.

The afflictions were discussed in the beginning of Chapter Two. The way to remove them is given in sutras 2.10 and 2.11. If the afflictions are weak, they are destroyed by returning to the original state, which is a state of awareness. If the afflictions are active or strong, they are destroyed through meditation. Similarly, if the identification with the mind and body is weak, it can be destroyed by returning to a state of awareness, or by being aware of the Self. If the identification is strong, it is destroyed through meditation. Once we reach a state of Samadhi, the mind has been stilled and we no longer identify with the mind, but only with the Self.

29

Prasaṁkhyāne 'py akusīdasya sarvathā viveka-khyāter dharma-meghaḥ samādhiḥ

When there is completely no interest in even profiteering from meditation, discriminating perception arises, which leads to Dharma-Megha (Shower of Virtue) Samadhi.

Patanjali has spent a considerable amount of time discussing the state of Samadhi. The first chapter is titled Samadhi. All of the first three chapters explain how we can reach a state of Samadhi. Samadhi is first without seed. Then, an impression arises which destroys all our other impressions, or our stock of karma, after which one attains seedless Samadhi. Patanjali has not said anywhere that seedless Samadhi is liberation. That is because one more step is required, which he explains here. Once we attain Samadhi, there is the possibility of gaining certain powers. This was explained in great detail in Chapter Three. One must not profit or personally benefit from these powers. Samadhi leads to liberation only if we have no interest in benefitting from these powers.

Once we have no interest in gaining from the spiritual powers, then discriminating perception arises, which removes our ignorance and leads to our liberation. Patanjali had discussed discriminating perception in Chapter Two, sutras 26 and 28. He said there that discriminating perception is the means for removing ignorance, and it arises by practicing the limbs of yoga. Normally, our perception is very limited. We are not able to see clearly and understand what is real and what is unreal. Imagine we are in a dark room. We are unable to see what is in the room. Suddenly, the light comes on and we are able to see everything. That is what discriminating perception is. It enhances our perception greatly. It removes the darkness of our ignorance and brings in the light of our liberation.

Dharma means law, duty, virtue, or justice. In this sutra it means virtue. Megha means shower, cloud, or multitude. Dharma-Megha Samadhi literally means, "Shower of Virtue" Samadhi. This is the state of liberation.

In the state of Samadhi, the activities of the mind have been stilled. The ego is almost completely gone. Therefore, there is very little chance of a person who has attained Samadhi, misusing the powers that are acquired in that state. To misuse powers, there has to be an ego present. Without an ego, why would one try and personally benefit from these powers? This is a natural check that Nature has kept on these powers. They are only obtained at a time when there is very little possibility of its misuse. Still, there has to be complete disinterest in profiteering from them, in order to be liberated.

30

Tataḥ kleśa-karma-nivṛttiḥ

From there, all afflictions and karmas disappear.

In the state of liberation all afflictions and karmas disappear. There are five afflictions that were mentioned in the beginning of Chapter Two—ignorance, egoism, attraction, aversion, and tenacity for mundane existence. Ignorance is the source of the subsequent afflictions. Once ignorance is removed, the other afflictions also disappear.

31

Tadā sarvāvaraṇa-malāpetasya
jñānasyānantyāj jñeyam alpam

Then, all coverings and impurities are removed and due to the infinity of knowledge gained, there is little left to be known.

After liberation, all coverings and impurities are removed and we are in a state of oneness with God. In that state, there is an infinity of knowledge gained and there is very little left to be known.

32

Tataḥ kṛtārthānāṁ
pariṇāma-krama-parisamāptir guṇānām

After that, the qualities of nature end their process of evolution, as their purpose has been accomplished.

The qualities of nature are a reference to the external physical world. The physical world is there for us to evolve and to be liberated. People enter our lives and events take place in our lives, to help us evolve. Be careful not to judge people or events, as you may not understand their true purpose. All events in our lives take place to help us in our process of evolution. It is the same with people who come into our lives. They are all there to assist us in our journey toward enlightenment.

The qualities of nature, or life, end the process of evolution for a liberated person because their purpose has been accomplished. That person has become liberated.

33

Kṣaṇa-pratiyogī
pariṇāmāparānta-nirgrāhyaḥ kramaḥ

This process of evolution is a series of moments, each dependent on the other, and is perceivable at the very end of the evolution.

Moments in our life move us forward in our evolution. Each moment is dependent on earlier moments. This process of evolution will only become completely clear to us, at the end of our evolution, when we are liberated. Then, we will look back at all the moments of our life and previous lives, and marvel at the beauty of it all. In the meantime, trust the process of life, or trust God, and understand that life is only on our side, helping us evolve.

34

Puruṣārtha-śūnyānāṁ guṇānāṁ pratiprasavaḥ kaivalyaṁ svarūpa-pratiṣṭhā vā citi-śakter iti

> **Therefore, liberation is the state where the qualities of nature, having no further purpose for the soul, return to their original state, Or, in other words, the energy of Consciousness settles in its own form.**

Patanjali ends by defining the state of *Kaivalya*, which is the state of liberation, or absolute oneness. It is the state where the qualities of nature, or the physical world, return to their original state as they have no further purpose for the soul. The original state is a non-physical state. He further says that this is a state where the energy of Consciousness settles in its own form. This is a non-dualistic way to describe ultimate reality. In dualism, the physical world or Nature, is separate from God. In non-dualism, Nature is the energy of God or Consciousness. There is no separation between Nature and God. In ultimate reality or *Kaivalya*, the energy of God returns to its own form.

Although written almost three thousand years ago, the message of the *Yoga Sutras* is as relevant today as it was three thousand years ago. Its wisdom is eternal. Patanjali explains so clearly how life works, what causes our suffering and the means to overcome our suffering. Our world has made great progress materially. Our lives are far more comfortable today, then they were even a hundred years ago. However, human suffering is still so prevalent. As Patanjali explained in the very second sutra of Chapter One—*Stilling the activities of the mind, is yoga.* There are two activities of the mind that cause the majority of our suffering—our imagination and our memory. Patanjali gives us so many ways to still our mind and reach a state of enlightenment. Our happiness does not depend on the amount of wealth we gather but on the amount of control we have over our minds. The more still our minds become, the greater is the peace and happiness we experience.

We can only bow down in gratitude to Patanjali, for his gift of the *Yoga Sutras.*

BIBLIOGRAPHY

Alladi, Krishnaswami. *Touched by the Goddess.* Available at: <https://inference-review.com/article/touched-by-the-goddess>

Batabyal, Rakesh. Noahkali: Where Gandhi waged the battle for India. Available at: <https://www.nationalheraldindia.com/india/noakhali-where-gandhi-waged-the-battle-for-india>

Brunton, Paul. A Search in Secret India. London: Rider, 1934, 2003.

Bryant, Edwin. F. *The Yoga Sutras of Patanjali.* USA: Macmillan, 2019.

Burtt, Edwin. A. *The Teachings of The Compassionate Buddha.* USA: New American Library, 1955, 1982.

Byrom, Thomas. *The Heart of Awareness—A Translation of the Ashtavakra Gita.* Boston: Shambhala, 1990, 2001.

Chakravarti, Sudeep. *Gandhi in Noakhali: The Bloody Battle for East Bengal.* Available at: <https://www.livehistoryindia.com/story/making-of-modern-india/gandhi-in-noakhali/>

Chaudhri, Ranjit. *112 Meditations for Self Realization: Vigyan Bhairava Tantra.* India: Prakash Books India Pvt. Ltd, 2011.

Chaudhri, Ranjit. *The Shiva Sutras: Eternal Wisdom for Life.* India: Prakash Books India Pvt. Ltd, 2019.

Chaudhri, Ranjit. *Sounds Of Liberation, The Spanda Karikas.* India: Prakash Books India Pvt. Ltd, 2021.

Dass, Ram. *Be Here Now.* USA: Lama Foundation, 1971, 1978.

Gandhi, M. K. *An Autobiography or The Story of My Experiments with Truth.* Penguin Books Ltd. 1927, 1982.

Gopalakrishnan, Dr. Sudha. *Abhinavagupta.* Available at: <https://www.sahapedia.org/abhinavagupta>

His Divine Grace A. C. Bhaktivedanta Swami Prabhupada. *Bhagavad Gita as It Is.* Mumbai: The Bhaktivedanta Book Trust, 1972, 2019.

India Today. *Srinivasa Ramanujan: The mathematical genius who credited his 3900 formulae to visions from Goddess Mahalakshmi.* Available at: <https://www.indiatoday.in/education-today/gk-current-affairs/story/srinivasa-ramanujan>

Katie, Byron. *Loving What Is: Four questions that can change your life.* New York: Three Rivers Press, 2002, 2003.

Lidke, Dr. Jeffrey. S. *A Thousand Years of Abhinavagupta.* Available at: <www.sutrajournal.com/a-thousand-years-of-abhinavagupta-by-jeffrey-lidke>

Maharaj, Sri Nisargadatta. *I Am That.* India: Chetana (P) Ltd, 1973, 2003.

Maharshi, Sri Ramana. *Words of Grace.* Tiruvannamalai: Sri Ramanasramam, 1969, 1996.

Mascaro, Juan. *The Bhagavad Gita.* England: Penguin Books Ltd, 1962, 1994.

Mascaro, Juan. *The Upanishads.* England: Penguin Books Ltd, 1965, 1981.

Mukherjee, Radhakamal. *Astavakragita* (The Song of the Self Supreme). India: Motilal Banarsidass Publishers Private Limited, 1971, 2000.

Radhakrishnan, S. *The Principal Upanishads.* India: Harper Collins Publishers India, 1994, 1997.

Razdan, Vinayak. *Abhinavagupta's cave, Beerwah, 1935.* Available at: <https://searchkashmir.org/2016/06/abhinavaguptas-cave-beerwah-1935.html>

Sadhguru. *How Adi Shankaracharya Entered a Dead King's Body.* Available at: <https://isha.sadhguru.org/in/en/wisdom/article/how-adishankara-entered-dead-king-body>

Sadhguru. *Karma, A Yogi's Guide to Crafting Your Destiny.* India: Penguin Ananda, 2021.

Sadhguru. *Death, An Inside Story.* India: Penguin Ananda, 2020.

Saraswati, Swami Satyananda. *Asana Pranayama Mudra Bandha.* India: Bihar School of Yoga, 1966, 1996.

Saraswati, Swami Satyananda. *Four Chapters on Freedom.* India: Bihar School of Yoga, 1976, 1989.

Sri Ramanasramam. *The Spiritual Teachings of Ramana Maharshi.* Boston: Shambhala Publications Inc, 1988.

Sunder, Kalpana. *The birthplace of Gandhi's peaceful protest.* Available at: <www.bbc.com/travel/story/20190325-the-birthplace-of-gandhis-peaceful-protest>

Sri Swami Satchidananda. *The Yoga Sutras of Patanjali.* USA: Integral Yoga Publications, 1978, 2020.

Swami Nikhilananda. *The Gospel of Sri Ramakrishna.* India: Sri Ramakrishna Math, 1996, 2019.

Swami Saradananda, translated by Swami Chetanananda. *Sri Ramakrishna and His Divine Play.* India: Vedanta Society of St. Louis, 2003, 2020.

Swami Vivekananda. *Raja Yoga: Conquering the Internal Nature.* India: Advaita Ashrama, 1923, 2000.

Swaminathan, Santanam. *Miracle of Entering into Another Body*! Available at: <https://www.speakingtree.in/blog/miracle-of-entering-in-to-another-body>

The Holy Bible, King James Version. New York: New American Library, 1974.

Tolle, Eckhart. *A New Earth: Awakening to Your Life's Purpose.* England: Penguin Books Ltd, 2005, 2006.

Tolle Eckhart. *The Power of Now: A Guide to Spiritual Enlightenment.* India: Yogi Impressions, 1997, 2001.

Venkataramiah, Mungala. *Talks with Sri Ramana Maharshi.* Tiruvannamalai: Sri Ramanasramam, 1955, 2000.

Walsch, Neale Donald. *Conversations With God Book 3, An uncommon dialogue.* Great Britain: Hodder and Stoughton, 1999.

Walsch, Neale Donald. *Conversations With God Book 4, Awaken the Species.* USA: Rainbow Ridge Books, 2017.

Walsch, Neale Donald. *Home with God, In A Life That Never Ends.* USA: Atria Books, 2006.

Walsch, Neale Donald. *Tomorrow's God: Our Greatest Spiritual Challenge.* USA: Atria Books, 2004.

White, David Gordon. *The Yoga Sutra of Patanjali.* USA: Princeton University Press, 2014, 2019.

Yogananda, Sri Sri Paramahansa. *God Talks with Arjuna: The Bhagavad Gita.* Kolkata: Yogoda Satsanga Society of India, 2002.

https://dailystoic.com

THE SUTRAS

CHAPTER ONE

SAMĀDHI PĀDA

SAMADHI

1. Now, instructions on yoga.
2. Stilling the activities of the mind, is yoga.
3. Then, the Seer abides in its own nature.
4. Otherwise, one identifies with the activities of the mind.
5. There are five types of activities of the mind, and these are either painful or pain-free.
6. They are right beliefs, wrong beliefs, imagination, sleep and memory.
7. The sources of right beliefs are direct experience, inference and authoritative scriptures.
8. Wrong beliefs are false knowledge that is not based on the true nature of something.
9. Knowledge resulting from words that are devoid of reality, is imagination.

10. Sleep is the activity, without the intellect as its foundation.

11. Past experiences remembered, is memory.

12. The activities of the mind are stilled by continuous practice and detachment.

13. Of the two, perseverance in effort is continuous practice.

14. And it becomes firmly established, when it is practiced uninterruptedly for a long time, with care and attention.

15. Detachment is that mastered state of consciousness, when one is not desirous of sense objects, whether experienced or heard.

16. Following that, due to perception of the soul, there is freedom from desires for the qualities of nature.

17. By extinguishing thinking, reflection, sensual enjoyment and egoism, one attains Samprajnata (Samadhi).

18. Through the continuous practice mentioned earlier, the intellect ceases and only the impressions remain. This is another way.

19. Yogis not identified with their bodies, attain this stilled state of being.

20. For others, Samprajnata Samadhi is preceded by faith, vigour and remembrance.

21. This is near for those with an intense desire for liberation.

22. That also depends on whether the intensity is weak, moderate or strong.

23. Or from service to God.

24. God is a special Soul, untouched by afflictions, actions, fruits of actions and the karmic process.

25. In God, is the source of omniscience that is unsurpassed.

26. Unbound by time, God is the Guru even for those who came before.

27. The sound expressing him is AUM.

28. Continuous recitation of it will manifest its meaning.

29. From this practice, consciousness turns inwards, and all obstacles are destroyed as well.

30. Disease, dullness, doubt, carelessness, laziness, intemperance, false perception, lack of depth in meditation and unsteadiness. These distractions of the mind are the obstacles.

31. Suffering, despair, trembling of the body and irregular breathing. These arise along with the distractions.

32. For preventing them, continuously practice on the one true element.

33. From being friendly toward the happy, compassionate toward the suffering, joyful to the virtuous and disregarding toward the wicked, brings about calmness of mind.

34. Or, by exhalation and retention of the breath.

35. Or, this state arises, through steadiness in fixing the mind on an object of sense.

36. Or, by focussing on the luminous Self within, that is untouched by sorrow.

37. Or, when the mind is free from attachment to any sense object.

38. Or, knowing that which supports the state of dreaming and deep sleep.

39. Or, by meditating on whatever is dear to one.

40. This yogi's mastery extends from the smallest particle to the end of the largest one.

41. Samapatti is the state when the activities of the mind have subsided and the mind becomes similar to a pure crystal, which reflects the colours of any object placed near it. In this state, the perceiver, the perceived object and the perceiving of it, appear one.

42. In that state, the distinction between the sound (perceiver), the object and the knowing of it, is all mixed up. This is Savitarka Samapatti.

43. When the memory is cleansed, it seems like one's own form is non-existent, and the object only appears. This is Nirvitarka (Samadhi).

44. By the same way, Savicara and Nirvicara, which are practiced on subtle objects, are explained.

45. And the subtleness of the object being meditated on, extends up to the imperceptible.

46. These are all in fact, Samadhi with seed (Sabija).

47. With expertise in Nirvicara, the Supreme Self shines.

48. That state carries divine truth, which is wisdom.

49. This wisdom because of its extraordinary sense, belongs to a different realm from the wisdom heard from scriptures, or from inference.

50. The impression produced by that state, destroys all other impressions.

51. On the destruction of even that impression, all impressions are destroyed, and one attains Nirbija (seedless) Samadhi.

CHAPTER TWO

SĀDHANA PĀDA

SPIRITUAL PRACTICE

1. Austerities, study of sacred scriptures and service to God, constitute Kriya Yoga.

2. Kriya Yoga is practiced for minimizing the afflictions and for bringing about Samadhi.

3. The afflictions are ignorance, egoism, attraction, aversion and tenacity of mundane existence.

4. Ignorance is the source of the subsequent afflictions, whether they are dormant, weak, intermittent or strong.

5. Ignorance is to perceive the transient as eternal, the impure as pure, pain as pleasure, and the non-self as the Self.

6. Egoism is identifying with the creation of the Seer—the instrument of experiencing (body and mind).

7. Being influenced by pleasure, is attraction.

8. Being influenced by pain, is aversion.

9. The tenacity of mundane existence flows by its own force. This is pervasive even amongst the wise.
10. If these afflictions are weak, they can be destroyed by returning to the original state.
11. If they are in an active state, they can be destroyed through meditation.
12. The storehouse of Karma has its root in these afflictions. The fruits of Karma (action) are experienced in the present and future lives.
13. As long as the root exists, the fruits of action result in birth as a particular kind, for a life span, and various experiences.
14. These experiences of pleasure and pain are consequences, caused by being virtuous or wicked.
15. To one of discrimination, everything is suffering in fact. This is due to the suffering that is latent in the impressions, the sorrow over changing circumstances and the inherent contradictions in the functioning of the qualities of nature.
16. Suffering that is yet to come, can be avoided.
17. The union of the Seer and the Seen, causes avoidance of this suffering.
18. The Seen consists of the sense organs and elements, and has the nature of inertia, activity and illumination. Its purpose is both, experiencing life and liberation of the soul.
19. The different stages of progression of the qualities of nature are non-physical, physical, indistinctive, and distinctive.
20. The Seer is nothing but the power of seeing. Although pure, it appears to perceive through the beliefs of the mind.
21. The Seen only exists for the liberation of the Self (Seer).

22. Once that purpose is accomplished, the Seen disappears for the liberated but it continues to exist for the others, being common for them all.

23. Realization of one's own nature is caused by the union of the Creator with its own energy (creation).

24. The cause of this union is ignorance.

25. From the absence of ignorance, no such union takes place. This is the state of absolute oneness of the Seer.

26. Uninterrupted discriminating perception is the means for its removal.

27. One's wisdom in the final stages is in seven parts.

28. By practicing the limbs of yoga, the impurities dissolve and the light of knowledge arises, culminating in discriminating perception.

29. The eight limbs of yoga are: Yama (self-disciplines), Niyama (observances), Asana (postures), Pranayama (breath practices), Pratyahara (sensory detachment), Dharana (concentration), Dhyana (meditation) and Samadhi.

30. The Yamas (self-disciplines) are non-violence, truthfulness, not stealing, being on the path of God and not having unnecessary possessions.

31. These great vows apply to the entire world, and are not limited by class, place, time or circumstances.

32. The Niyamas (observances) are cleanliness, contentment, austerities, study of sacred texts and service to God.

33. On being disturbed by negative thoughts, think of their opposite.

34. When these negative thoughts such as violence, etc. are acted on and performed, or caused to be performed, or agreed upon, they are preceded by greed, anger or delusion, which may be weak, moderate or strong. The consequences of these acts of ignorance, is endless suffering. Therefore, think of opposite thoughts, when negative thoughts arise.

35. In the presence of one who is established in non-violence, all enmity ceases.

36. A person established in truthfulness, receives the fruits of their actions.

37. For one established in not stealing, all wealth approaches.

38. A person established on the path of God, gains vigour.

39. On perseverance of, not having unnecessary possessions, one obtains complete knowledge of the 'how and why' of birth.

40. From cleanliness, one develops a distaste for one's own body and for comingling with other bodies.

41. And one develops purity of nature, cheerfulness, one pointedness, control over the senses and readiness for Self-Realization.

42. From Contentment, unsurpassed happiness is obtained.

43. From practicing austerities, the impurities are removed, and the body and sense organs reach a state of perfection.

44. From the study of sacred scriptures, arises union with one's favourite deity.

45. From service to God, comes complete attainment of Samadhi.

46. Asana is a stable and comfortable posture.

47. By both, hardly moving and joining with the eternal.

48. Thereafter, one is not afflicted by the dualities.

49. After that stable posture is maintained, regulate the flow of breath—inhalation and exhalation. This is Pranayama (breath practices).

50. The movement of the breath is either external, internal or stationary. It is regulated by part, time and number, and is either long or short.

51. The fourth type is beyond the limits of the external and the internal.

52. Thereafter, the covering over the inner light, is destroyed.

53. And the mind becomes fit for concentration.

54. When the senses detach from their own objects, they seem to resemble the mind's own form. This is Pratyahara (sensory detachment).

55. Then, there is complete control over the senses.

CHAPTER THREE

VIBHŪTI PĀDA

SPIRITUAL POWERS

1. Concentration is fixing the mind to one place or object.
2. Meditation is the continuous flow of attention, on that place or object.
3. That same meditation, when only the object appears and it seems like one's own form is non-existent, that is Samadhi.
4. These three practiced together, is Samyama.
5. From mastery of Samyama, comes the light of wisdom.
6. Its application is to be done in stages.
7. These three—Concentration, Meditation and Samadhi, are internal limbs, compared to the preceding limbs.
8. However, these three are external limbs, of the seedless Samadhi.
9. The appearance of the overpowering impression, which destroys all other impressions, occurs the

moment after the mind is stilled. This development takes place on stilling the activities of the mind.

10. Its extinguishment is activated by that impression.

11. On diminishment in thinking of many things, and rise in one-pointedness of the mind, there is development in Samadhi.

12. Then again, when the idea that has passed and that which has arisen is the same, that is development of one-pointedness of the mind.

13. Through this, the transformations in the nature, qualities and conditions of the elements and the senses, is also fully explained.

14. A living being with its individual characteristics, has a past, present and future, with its nature and qualities determined as a consequence of the preceding stage.

15. The difference in these successive stages is the cause of the difference in evolution.

16. From Samyama on the three transformations (of nature, qualities and conditions), knowledge of the past and future is obtained.

17. A sound, its meaning and the idea of it, are sometimes superimposed on each other, causing confusion. By performing Samyama on them separately, knowledge of the speech of all living beings is obtained.

18. By doing Samyama directly on the impressions, one gains knowledge of previous births.

19. From Samyama on their beliefs, one gains knowledge of another's mind.

20. But that does not include the motives as that is not the object of the Samyama.

21. From Samyama on the form of one's body, one gains the ability to stop being perceived by others, by stopping light being reflected (from the body) to their eyes, and one becomes invisible.

22. By this way, the disappearance of sound, etc, is also explained.

23. Karma is either manifesting or is dormant. From Samyama on these Karmas, or from portents of death, one obtains knowledge of one's death.

24. By Samyama on friendliness, etc, powers are gained.

25. From Samyama on strengths, the strength of an elephant, etc, are gained.

26. From Samyama on the light of perception within, one acquires knowledge of the small, the concealed and the distant.

27. From Samyama on the sun, knowledge of the world is gained.

28. From performing Samyama on the moon, knowledge of the arrangement of the stars, is acquired.

29. By Samyama on the pole star, knowledge of the movement of the stars is obtained.

30. From Samyama on the navel chakra, knowledge of the arrangement of the body is gained.

31. From Samyama on the pit of the throat, hunger and thirst cease.

32. From Samyama on the tortoise shaped channel, stability is obtained.

33. From Samyama on the light at the top of the head, visions of realized masters are obtained.

34. Or from Divine intuition, comes everything.

35. From Samyama on the heart, knowledge of the mind is acquired.

36. The mind and the Self are completely different from each other. The belief that they are the same, is the cause of our experience. The mind exists for the Self. From Samyama on that which exists for itself (the Self), knowledge of the Self is obtained.

37. From this, Divine intuition, hearing, touch, vision and smell, are born.

38. On awakening, these powers are obstacles in Samadhi.

39. From loosening the instrument of connection with one's body and by knowing the process of the mind, one may enter another person's body.

40. From mastery over the *Udana* life energy, the body can levitate, and one can walk over water, mud, thorns, etc, without touching them.

41. From mastery over Samana life energy, one becomes radiant.

42. From Samyama on the relationship between the ear and space, one is able to listen to Divine sounds.

43. From Samyama on the relationship between the body and space, and from Samapatti on the lightness of cotton, one acquires the ability to travel through space.

44. Practice Samyama on the great liberated souls, who are in their natural state. Thereafter, the covering over the inner light is removed.

45. Our own gross form is constructed from the subtle elements. From Samyama on their significance, one gains mastery over the elements.

46. After that, *Anima* and other powers appear, the body attains perfection and there is no damage to its essential quality.

47. Grace, beauty, strength, toughness, and robustness, comprise perfection of the body.

48. The grasping quality of one's nature follows from egoism. From Samyama on its significance, one gains mastery over the senses.

49. From that, comes speed like the mind, existence, independent of the senses and mastery over primary matter.

50. Only for one who perceives the difference between the mind and the Self, does the state of omnipotence and omniscience arise.

51. From detachment to even that, the seed of deficiency is destroyed, and one attains liberation.

52. On receiving an invitation from celestial beings for intercourse, one should not accept, nor be proud as there is the possibility of falling back into the undesirable.

53. From Samyama on a moment and its successive moments, comes knowledge arising from discrimination.

54. From seeing no separable difference by race, attributes, or part, compared to two objects of the same kind, arises knowledge.

55. This knowledge arising from discrimination, is liberating. It covers all regions and all objects and happens in an instant.

56. When the purity of the mind becomes equal to that of the Self, there is liberation.

CHAPTER FOUR

KAIVAḶYA PĀDA

LIBERATION

1. The spiritual powers arise from birth, herbs, mantras, austerities, or Samadhi.

2. The change into a different kind at birth, is for satisfying the desires of one's nature.

3. The motive is not the cause of nature choosing a particular kind, but then, it acts like a cultivator.

4. Minds are created entirely from ego.

5. There is one mind of the many, that is responsible for the manifestation of variety.

6. Among them, those born from meditation have no stock of karma.

7. The actions of a yogi are neither white nor black. For the others, it is of three kinds.

8. Thereafter, the consequences of past actions, stored as impressions, will manifest only at a suitable time.

9. Though separated by birth, place and time, there is continuity because memory and impressions are the same in form.

10. The impressions have no beginning because desires have been in existence for eternity.

11. The impressions are held together and sustained through the interconnectedness between the motive for an action and its consequence. On their disappearance, the impressions also disappear.

12. The past and the future exist in their own form. This is due to a break into parts, in the journey of the established order of things.

13. Whether manifested or unmanifested, they have the qualities of the Self.

14. The reality of objects is due to their transformation from oneness.

15. Due to the mind dividing the sameness of objects, the path of these two appears different.

16. And nor does an object's existence depend on a single mind. Otherwise, what would be the proof of that object, in its absence?

17. An object is known or unknown, depending on the mind's colouring of it.

18. The activities of the mind are always known to its master, the soul, due to the soul's unchanging nature.

19. Nor is the mind self-illuminating because it is an instrument of the soul.

20. And it cannot know both simultaneously.

21. One mind being an object of another mind, would imply one intellect governing another, which is unworkable. And there would also be a mixing up of memory.
22. When there is no intermixing of thoughts; when that state of mind appears, one's own intelligence becomes known.
23. The mind that is coloured by the Seer and the Seen, knows everything.
24. However, the mind with its varied and innumerable latent impressions, exists for the sake of another (the soul) because it can only act by being in contact with it.
25. For one who sees the difference between the mind and the Self, the idea of the mind being the Self, disappears.
26. Then, the mind becomes inclined toward discrimination and is close to liberation.
27. During breaks in that state, other ideas may arise due to latent impressions.
28. These can be removed just like the afflictions, explained earlier.
29. When there is completely no interest in even profiteering from meditation, discriminating perception arises, which leads to Dharma-Megha (Shower of Virtue) Samadhi.
30. From there, all afflictions and karmas disappear.
31. Then, all coverings and impurities are removed and due to the infinity of knowledge gained, there is little left to be known.
32. After that, the qualities of nature end their process of evolution, as their purpose has been accomplished.

33. This process of evolution is a series of moments, each dependent on the other, and is perceivable at the very end of the evolution.

34. Therefore, liberation is the state where the qualities of nature, having no further purpose for the soul, return to their original state, Or, in other words, the energy of Consciousness settles in its own form.

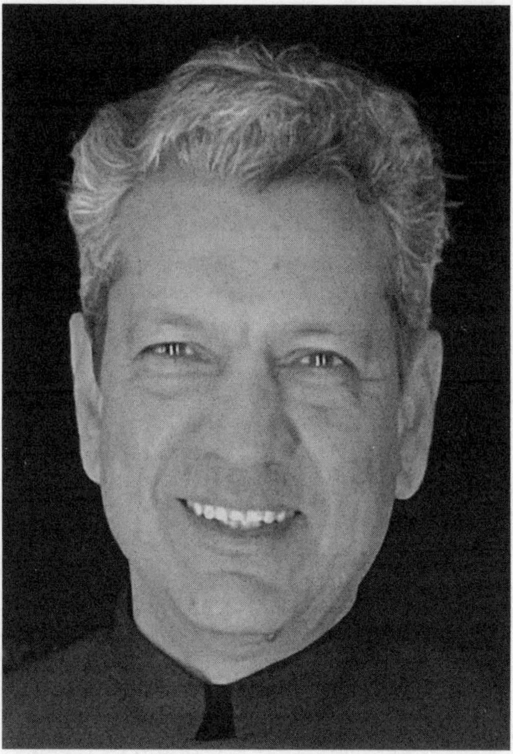

ABOUT THE AUTHOR

Ranjit Chaudhri is a national bestselling author who has translated some important texts of Yoga and Kashmir Shaivism from Sanskrit to English. These include *The Shiva Sutras: Eternal Wisdom for Life, 112 Meditations for Self Realization: The Vigyan Bhairava Tantra,* and *Sounds of Liberation: The Spanda Karikas.* He believes the wisdom of some of our ancient spiritual texts can lead to self-transformation and make the world a better place. His extensive knowledge of yoga, gained from over forty years of experience, helps to explain, and clarify the profound messages of the texts he has translated. He presently lives in Kolkata.